*MAKING THE PATIENT
YOUR PARTNER*

MAKING THE PATIENT YOUR PARTNER

Communication Skills for Doctors and Other Caregivers

THOMAS GORDON, Ph.D., AND
W. STERLING EDWARDS, M.D.

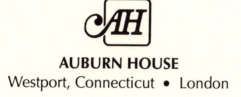

AUBURN HOUSE
Westport, Connecticut • London

Library of Congress Cataloging-in-Publication Data

Gordon, Thomas.
    Making the patient your partner : communication skills for
doctors and other caregivers / Thomas Gordon and W. Sterling Edwards.
        p.   cm.
    Includes bibliographical references and index.
    ISBN 0–86569–255–6 (alk. paper)
    1. Medical personnel and patient.   2. Interpersonal communication.
3. Communication in medicine.   I. Edwards, W. Sterling.
II. Title.
    [DNLM: 1. Professional-Patient Relations.   2. Interpersonal
Relations.   3. Communication.   W 62 G665m 1995]
    R727.3.G63   1995
    610.69′6—dc20
    DNLM/DLC
    for Library of Congress   94–42698

British Library Cataloguing in Publication Data is available.

Library of Congress Catalog Card Number: 94–42698
ISBN: 0–86569–255–6

First published in 1995

Auburn House, 88 Post Road West, Westport, CT 06881
An imprint of Greenwood Publishing Group, Inc.

Printed in the United States of America

The paper used in this book complies with the
Permanent Paper Standard issued by the National
Information Standards Organization (Z39.48–1984).

10 9 8 7 6 5 4 3 2 1

Copyright Acknowledgment

The authors and publisher gratefully acknowledge permission for use of the following material:

Extracts from P. Bellet and M. Maloney, "The Importance of Empathy as an Interviewing Skill in Medicine," *JAMA*, 266, 1991, pp. 1831–1832. Copyright © 1991, American Medical Association.

Every reasonable effort has been made to trace the owners of copyright materials in this book, but in some instances this has proven impossible. The authors and publisher will be glad to receive information leading to more complete acknowledgments in subsequent printings of the book and in the meantime extend their apologies for any omissions.

Contents

Preface

This book is written for all health professionals who relate directly to patients, such as doctors, nurses, psychologists, hospital chaplains, and social workers. It is also a book for all others who give care to the ill: hospital and hospice volunteers, nursing home personnel, spouses, families, and friends. The focus of the book is on improving the way such persons communicate with patients.

The authors have come to believe that it is possible for caregivers, both professional and nonprofessional, to help the sick person feel respected, supported, and trusted at every stage of the patient's illness—whether that critical first visit to the physician's office, the emotional anguish when submitting to various diagnostic procedures, extended confinement in a hospital, a prolonged struggle with a life-threatening illness, or facing the inevitability of death.

In spite of the tremendous medical advances that have been made in the 20th century, there are still many illnesses that cannot be "cured" by medical means and some that can only be controlled by lifelong treatment. It is disappointing that medicine seems to have made little progress, or, as some believe, even to have gone backward in dealing with the emotional components of serious illness. The old family doctor had an image of being more empathic than the modern medical specialist, but perhaps this was because empathy was the main tool he had. Only now are we beginning to realize how valuable that emotional support can be.

Countless studies have shown that a large percentage of patients become dissatisfied with their relationships with health professionals. And the source of that dissatisfaction is seldom the technical incompetence of the health professional. More often it is the ineffectiveness of the communication between them. Most patients don't feel encouraged to ask questions or talk about all that's bothering them, and they are often unclear about what the health professional tells them. Research studies employing tape recordings of the medical interview show frequent interruptions of patients and little empathy.

For the nonprofessional caregivers—spouses, families, friends—a serious illness is almost as disruptive as if they were the patient. Beginning with the onset of symptoms and the diagnosis, there is anxiety and fear of the unknown. Most people have no experience coping with the emotional changes in the patient, let alone recognizing and dealing with their own feelings. And most laypeople don't have the necessary communication skills to help patients talk about their problems or openly express their feelings.

The intent of the authors of this book is not to condemn or blame either health professionals or nonprofessional caregivers, for we recognize that inadequate interpersonal communication is also the rule rather than the exception with parents, teachers, lawyers, managers, salespeople, and almost any other group you can think of. This is because only recently has interpersonal communication become a field of study for social scientists and medical researchers. Their studies have clearly identified specific communication skills that strengthen relationships and those that weaken them. Certain kinds of talk can actually be therapeutic—helping people deal constructively with their negative emotions, find solutions to their problems, take control of their lives.

These "helping skills" can be particularly useful for *anyone* relating to patients. The authors found abundant research evidence showing that patients who experience effective two-way communication with their health professional are more satisfied with their treatment, less inclined to initiate a malpractice suit, recover more quickly from surgery, and more likely to comply with the physician's treatment regime.

Nurses, social workers, hospice volunteers, and hospital chaplains are sometimes more attuned to the patient's feelings than are physicians. However, many of them are not aware that certain often-used verbal messages can be roadblocks to patients' communication, and that there are new and more effective ways to enhance relationships with patients.

It is possible for caregivers, both professional and nonprofessional to learn how to help the sick find peace, hope, and meaning in life regardless of the course of the physical part of the illness. Relationships with patients can become like a partnership with mutual support, respect, and trust.

The first chapter of the book provides evidence for the frequency of patients' dissatisfaction with their relationships with health professionals. It also documents the widespread recognition of this problem by physicians themselves and identifies the potential benefits to be derived from better communication between physicians and patients.

Chapters 2–6 and 12 were written by Dr. Gordon, who first makes a strong case for health professionals to adopt a new "relationship model" that is less paternalistic and more collaborative. Then Dr. Gordon presents the communication skills needed to build such relationships. These critical interpersonal skills are illustrated by interactions and dialogues, primarily between patients and their doctors or nurses.

Chapters 7–11, written by Dr. Edwards, focus on the special problems and needs of patients with chronic and life-threatening illnesses, and then illustrate the use of the interpersonal communication skills in relating to such patients. In these chapters the communication skills are illustrated by interactions and dialogues primarily between patients and those persons who most often care for them—such as hospice volunteers, counselors, nursing home personnel, spouses, family members, friends, and other caregivers.

Every one of us may become a caregiver at some point for a family member or a friend who is ill. The authors hope this book will be of help not only to health professionals but also to those caregivers who would like to empower patients to deal more constructively with their pain, their loneliness, their fears, and hopes.

Introduction

Thomas Gordon, Ph.D.

For 40 years my principal professional activity has been trying to identify the key interpersonal communication skills that foster satisfying and healthy relationships, and then developing effective ways to teach them to others.

My training in client-centered psychotherapy and a long association with its innovator, Carl Rogers, convinced me that the professional therapist's chief therapeutic tool, empathic and nonjudgmental "reflection of feelings," would be valuable to other professionals, such as teachers, clergy, personnel counselors, social workers—any member of a "helping profession." However, it was not until later, when I served as a psychological consultant to an industrial organization, that I discovered that this potent therapeutic skill could also be learned and utilized by managers and supervisors to foster better two-way communication with workers and build close and productive relationships with them.

This consulting experience launched me into a period of doing leadership training, during which I was to learn that other communication skills besides empathic listening were necessary for leaders to create a "therapeutic climate" for their group members. One of these interpersonal skills was authentic and nonevaluative self-disclosure—being open, honest, and direct in communicating thoughts, feelings, and concerns to others. I coined the term "I-Message" for this essential skill. Another skill leaders needed was group-centered problem-solving—getting workers to participate actively with their leader in solving work-related problems or setting rules and policies.

These early leadership training experiences influenced me to write my first book, *Group-Centered Leadership: A Way of Releasing the Creative Power of Groups.* Unfortunately, neither my colleagues nor many organizations were open to this collaborative and democratic model of leadership, which 20 years later would be called "participative management" and be widely taught in business schools and used by most of the Fortune 500 companies.

My next application of these critical interpersonal skills was in parent–child relationships. I designed a brief eight-session course and called it Parent Effectiveness Training (P.E.T.). I authorized other instructors to teach it, and within 10 years several thousand instructors were teaching P.E.T. in every state. As of this writing P.E.T. is taught in 37 countries, and well over a million persons have learned empathic listening (now called Active Listening), I-Messages, participative problem-solving and a fourth skill, called No-Lose Conflict Resolution.

By now, the benefits of these skills have been confirmed by a large body of research. The P.E.T. course alone has been evaluated in 60 or more research studies. Even more gratifying is the fact that my organization, Effectiveness Training International, coordinates a worldwide network of several thousand instructors teaching parents, leaders, teachers, clergy, social workers, counselors, nurses, and doctors.

Some years ago, Dr. Richard Feinbloom, a Harvard-trained pediatrician and author of the *Child Health Encyclopedia*, delivered an invited lecture at our national convention of Effectiveness Training instructors. His words were prophetic:

> There is a growing challenge to the disease model of illness. . . . Under what I call the facilitative model of medical practice, the doctor and patient are each persons in their own right, each with different information. The patient is a full partner in the management of his illness. . . . The doctor can increase the chances of being used as a consultant if he can first ally himself with the emotional needs of the patient through the process which you call Active Listening. . . . Thus the professional must increasingly become interested in how to help someone change his attitudes and modify his behavior. These goals require a far different set of skills than those traditionally taught in medical schools, which emphasize the diagnosis and treatment of disease.

It took Dr. W. Sterling Edwards, my coauthor, to resurrect my early interest in sharing with health professionals and other patient caregivers these remarkably effective interpersonal skills. Impressed with his innovative counseling of patients experiencing life-threatening diseases, I agreed to collaborate with him in writing a book that would use our combined experience to help both professionals and nonprofessionals improve the way they relate to patients.

Introduction
W. Sterling Edwards, M.D.

As I finished my medical training in the early '50s, my interest developed in cardiovascular surgery. What an exciting time to be involved in the exploding field of surgery of the heart and blood vessels. I was fortunate to be a part of the early development of artificial arteries of cloth and the correction of birth defects in the hearts of children. I thoroughly enjoyed teaching medical students and surgical residents, and treating the physical aspects of patients' illnesses. But I realize now that I didn't do a very good job of relating to patients whose conditions were beyond my technical skills to cure. I didn't know what to say, my visits were short, my conversations were superficial.

When our children left home, my wife went back to college, got a master's degree in guidance and counseling, and started a counseling practice. In the early 1970s she registered for a 17-day workshop in psychotherapy, and I decided to go along. There I met and was assigned to a small group under Carl Rogers, a pioneer in humanistic psychology. I was impressed by his emphasis on the client-centered approach to treatment of emotional problems, where the patient participated actively in decisions about her or his treatment. At about this time I was appointed chairman of the Surgery Department at the University of New Mexico School of Medicine and director of its surgical residents' training program. As a result of my exposure to Rogerian principles, I decided to see if it was possible to develop a humanistic surgical residency program in contrast to the "Marine boot camp" process of most programs. We developed a "resident-centered approach" where residents participated actively in decisions about their own learning. It worked. The morale was terrific, not only on the part of the residents but on the part of the faculty as well. Applications for the program multiplied. The humanistic aspect of the program became known all over the United States.

In 1987, I retired from surgery and from my teaching responsibilities at the university. In searching for a productive retirement career, I found myself attracted to psychology and the study of the emotional side of illness. I attended several courses in health psychology and some weekend psychology workshops. A number of nonmedical friends in recent years had developed life-threatening illnesses: cancer, heart disease, neurological problems. I began to ask these individuals if there was anything missing in their relationships with their professional and nonprofessional caregivers. A frequent answer was that caregivers of all kinds—doctors, nurses, family, friends—wanted to give information or advice, and very few wanted to listen to their feelings of fear, uncertainty, depression. That prompted me to explore the literature on listening.

This led to my discovery of the three best-selling books by Thomas Gordon, Ph.D., who had successfully taught hundreds of thousands of people a skill he called Active Listening. The three books on parent, teacher, and leader effectiveness training described how Active Listening and other communication skills could help individuals talk about their problems and express their feelings—often delving deeper and deeper into their own problems and often discovering solutions that were much better than others could ever advise. I decided to see if I could develop a "listening" practice for individuals with progressive or life-threatening illnesses. I also started a men's support group, a retired physicians' group, and a cancer patient support group.

In my individual counseling, I visit patients on referral, at their homes, at the hospital, or at the hospice unit. My objective is to encourage them to talk about their feelings about their illness or their relationships. I simply act as a listener, not judging or giving advice. I do this on a voluntary basis, since I want my relationship to be that of a friend rather than that of a professional. I make no diagnoses, give no second opinions, write no prescriptions. This experience has been tremendously fulfilling for me. I do not follow every patient until he or she dies. If I do not feel anticipation before a visit, fulfillment after the visit, and some connection during the visit, I am not getting any healing, and neither is the patient, so we break off by mutual consent.

After four years' experience I was encouraged by participants in several of these groups to write down my learnings in a small book. Since I had learned so much from the books of Thomas Gordon, I wrote to him and asked if he thought there was a need for a book to help caregivers become more effective and, if so, whether he would be interested in helping write one. I received an enthusiastic positive reply to both questions. So we set out to work together.

In working with Dr. Gordon, I learned there is a lot more to effective caregiving than just listening to patients. Active Listening does help when the patient has a problem, but what can be done to help when the patient is creating a disturbing problem for the caregiver? When is Active Listening inappropriate? What should a caregiver do if there is conflict and both have a problem? I learned that confrontive "I-Messages" and a six-step conflict resolution method, as taught in Tom's Effectiveness Training books and workshops, can be applied to the caregiver/patient relationship with great improvement in the quality of that relationship.

My own skills as a caregiver have greatly improved since my days as a surgeon. In this book Tom Gordon and I share our experiences with the reader.

MAKING THE PATIENT
YOUR PARTNER

Chapter 1

Dissatisfaction with Doctor-Patient Relationships

The doctor-patient relationship can be restored. But it will take commitment by people on both ends of the stethoscope.
—C. Everett Koop, M.D., *Koop*

Even with the incredible scientific and technological advances available to health professionals, communication still is seen as the core clinical procedure for diagnosing, treating, and caring for patients. Furthermore, patients' satisfaction with the way they are treated by health professionals is strongly influenced by the quality of the communication that occurs between them.

Literally hundreds of research studies have confirmed what most patients have actually experienced firsthand—that how they are talked to by health professionals and how well they feel understood by them determines the degree of their satisfaction with those relationships. And, most important, if patients are dissatisfied with those relationships, studies show that it can seriously reduce their compliance with (or adherence to) their treatment regimen, it can make them have serious doubts about the competence of their physician, it can negatively affect how long it takes to get well, and it can increase the frequency of patient malpractice suits.

Undoubtedly, health professionals sincerely want to develop and maintain good relationships with patients. However, like most members of other professions—attorneys, engineers, executives, dentists, teachers, clergy, architects, accountants, for example—health professionals have seldom been given adequate training in the interpersonal skills needed to create mutually satisfying and lasting relationships. In fact, the basic theory and methodology of interpersonal skill training is still in its infancy, with its origins dating back no earlier than the early 1950s. Only in recent years have some medical and nursing schools introduced such training for their students.

Not only has research shown that many patients are not satisfied with the quality of communication with health professionals, but even health professionals themselves—particularly physicians and nurses—recognize that there are serious problems in relations with patients. Prominent physicians have spoken out for humanizing the practice of medicine. Some have brought back the image of the old-fashioned family doctor as an ideal model for dealing with the emotional aspects of illness and for being more empathic with their patients. More recently, major professional medical societies have urgently called for more comprehensive training of doctors and medical students in interviewing and dealing with patients' "illness" as well as their "disease." Some of these professional groups have initiated their own training workshops for their members.

Based upon our combined experiences, we believe our book can make some important contributions to this growing movement for improving relationships between health professionals and patients. Each of us has received training in the communication skills deemed necessary and effective in creating interpersonal relationships that are mutually satisfying as well as therapeutic.

One of us (WSE) received his training with a group of other physicians in a workshop with psychologist Carl Rogers, renowned for developing client-centered psychotherapy, a method that relies heavily on empathic listening skills (Rogers, 1951). Using this training, he has been an empathic counselor for many patients, especially those with life-threatening diseases.

The other coauthor (TG), also a graduate student of Carl Rogers and later his faculty colleague at the University of Chicago, is widely recognized as a pioneer in the field of interpersonal skills training, beginning with a training program for organizational leaders (Leader Effectiveness Training) and later training for parents (Parent Effectiveness Training) and teachers (Teacher Effectiveness Training). These courses have trained over a million persons in 37 countries.

In this chapter we will provide some of the research evidence for patient dissatisfaction with physicians and other health professionals. We will also document the awareness of health professionals themselves of the dehumanization of patients. We will then identify the benefits that studies have shown will result from improved relationships with patients.

PATIENT DISSATISFACTION

Patient complaints about their relationships with health professionals are quite widespread.

Surveys on the frequency of patient dissatisfaction with health professionals have typically shown high percentages (Gerrard et al., 1980). Also alarming to some members of the medical profession is the increasingly widespread public opinion that the primary motivation of many physicians is monetary gain, not the benefit of the patient (Spencer, 1990).

Patients report that they often do not know the meaning of words used by doctors and nurses, so they fail to understand what they are told and are reluctant to ask for further information even when they would like to. Patients get interrupted within an average of 18 seconds of starting to tell their story or ask questions (Beckman and Frankel, 1984).

One study has shown that one-third of patients visiting the medical clinics of a large university hospital complained that their physicians did not pay enough attention to their ideas about treating their medical problems (Brody, 1980).

In her book *In the Patient's Best Interest: Women and the Politics of Medical Decisions*, Sue Fisher describes this incident.

> On my initial visit with the gynecologist, a nurse called me into an examining room, asked me to undress, gave me a paper bag to put on and told me the doctor would be with me soon. I was stunned. Was I not even to see the doctor before undressing? . . . How could I present myself as a competent, knowledgeable person sitting undressed on the examining table? But I had a potentially cancerous growth, so I did as I was told. . . . In a few minutes the nurse returned and said, "Lie down, the doctor is coming." Again I complied. The doctor entered the examining room, nodded in my direction while reading my chart and proceeded to examine me without ever having spoken to me. (Fisher, 1986, p. 2)

Another patient, herself a physician, writes about her experiences with her doctors when she had breast cancer.

Oncologists, radiation oncologists, plastic surgeons. . . . No one understood that I wasn't a statistic, that this was my life and that these were awful decisions. I resented the fact that they could just go home to their lives, whereas I still had cancer. My doctors gave me plenty of information but rarely took care of me. They knew how to cut into an anesthetized body, calculate radiation dosages and give statistics, but they weren't good at asking me how I was feeling. They barely acknowledged that I was a new mother and never mentioned what an absolutely overwhelming experience this must be. No one even gave me an affectionate pat, let alone a hug. Maybe they weren't trained to do this. Possibly they had been trained out of doing this. But what I needed doesn't really take training; it just takes being human. (Olmstead, 1993, p. 131)

The dissatisfaction of patients can manifest itself in various ways—noncompliance with treatment instructions; malpractice litigation; and the use of nontraditional health care providers such as acupuncturists, hypnotists, massage therapists, chiropractors, all of whom are often perceived as more interested in the patient as a person.

RECOGNITION OF THE PROBLEMS BY HEALTH PROFESSIONALS

In recent years particularly, some medical practitioners have warned their colleagues of the trend away from the "treatment of the human being" and the "commitment to the patient." In describing their concept of the ideal role of the physician, some use the term "humanistic health model" and contrast it with "technological soldier." Others recommend moving from a "problem focus" to a "person focus"; others see an unfortunate trend away from the physician's warm bedside manner—away from the model of the old-fashioned general practitioner. Some see the problem as a trend away from the physician as a compassionate helper or the Good Samaritan. Still others define the problem in medicine as one of treatment being too much physician-centered and not enough patient-centered. Others regret that physicians are forgetting the art of medicine.

Dr. C. Everett Koop, former surgeon general, addresses "the spiritual aspects of health care," stressing that health care professionals have a spiritual heritage of cherishing life. However, "We put too much emphasis on *curing*, especially when a disease is fatal, and not enough on *caring* . . .

curing costs millions but caring comes from the heart and soul. I hope Americans never run out of either" (Koop, 1992, p. 5).

Pediatrician Naomi Remen, writing under the auspices of the Institute for the Study of Humanistic Medicine, saw another kind of trend.

> During the past 50 years, the art of medicine has gradually become separated from the science of medicine. Modern physicians increasingly tend to serve their patients with science alone. But while patients acknowledge the value of scientific care, they are increasingly more discontent, more critical and even more hostile about their medical care than ever before. (Remen, 1975, p. 2)

Other medical historians perceive that the profession of medicine has lost its strong motivation to help fellow human beings in distress. They recognize that the high status the profession earned was based for centuries almost entirely on treating patients as human beings. However, as scientific advances proliferated in the 20th century, it is widely believed that concentrating on treating the disease has come to predominate over treating the illness of the patient.

In his 1990 Presidential Address to the American College of Surgeons, Frank C. Spencer strongly calls for more humanism in the practice of medicine:

> Medicine originated with the fundamental human instinct to help a fellow human being in distress, the sympathy of man for man. The central importance of humanism is best understood by the fact that *the high status of medicine for centuries was based almost totally on humanism*. Today—in 1990—the vast majority of medicine is based on science, treating the disease that is present. (Spencer, 1990, p. 2)

Spencer added that eight other Presidential Addresses had echoed the same theme.

It is also widely recognized that nursing has become less patient-oriented and more scientifically oriented. Nurses now get more deeply involved with the *technology* of care—they often need to deal with complex machinery and excessive paperwork, which can distract them from some of their caring functions, the very activities that attracted them to the nursing profession in the first place.

Psychologist M. Robin DiMatteo describes this change that has taken place in the role of nurses—from being the main provider of care and

support of patients' physical and emotional needs to the more limited role
of helper to the physician:

> In such environments many nurses become highly dissatisfied with
> what they have been taught in school about taking care of patients and
> what they are able to do in practice. Many nurses are now seeking
> work environments that allow them more autonomy in caring for
> patients. . . . Like physicians, senior nursing students become more
> disease-oriented than patient-centered as time goes on, and over the
> course of training they spend less and less time meeting patients'
> nonmedical needs. (DiMatteo, 1991, p. 260)

Nothing has publicized the difficulties experienced by patients in their
relationship with physicians more widely than the movie *The Doctor*, a
story about the trying experiences of a physician who became a patient with
a malignant tumor on his vocal cords. The movie portrayed a doctor who
didn't understand the problems of patients until he was the patient himself
and had to give control of his life over to others and suffer some indignities.

SOME RELEVANT RESEARCH FINDINGS

The medical literature contains a large number of research studies that
have evaluated physician–patient interactions and documented the undesirable results of ineffective communication in such interviews.

Many date the beginning of research on doctor–patient communication
to the mid-60s, when Dr. Barbara Korsch installed video cameras into her
pediatric clinic examining rooms. As she then described her pioneering
work, "People were shocked that I was studying the hallowed doctor–patient relationship. It was like going into church with a video camera." Dr.
Korsch and her colleagues tape-recorded over 800 visits and later interviewed the mothers.

The tapes revealed that the interviews were "technical and information-
oriented." Everyday civilities such as greetings and handshakes were seldom used, expressions of friendliness were rare, and many of the mothers
felt tense and fearful. Nearly a quarter of the mothers said they were not
given a chance to bring up the one problem most on their minds. One out
of five felt they weren't given a clear explanation of what was wrong with
their child. Almost half were left unsure of what had caused the illness
(Korsch and Negrete, 1972).

A more recent study found that in encounters lasting 20 minutes, doctors spent just a little over a minute giving information to their patients. On the average, the doctors overestimated the time they spent giving information by about *a factor of nine.* In medical school and in their residency training, physicians learn to ask many questions in taking medical histories, yet the interrogative mode in a subtle way communitcates, "I am in charge here." Physicians who ask many questions are keeping tight control over the relationship. No wonder so many patients complain that the doctor doesn't listen to them. Researchers have concluded that "in doctor-patient encounters there is a dispreference for patient initiated questions," which reinforces the "high control style" that is so commonly used by physicians (Waitzkin, 1984).

One way that improvement of treatment can be realized by physicians is through increasing patient compliance (or cooperation) with the physician's orders. Estimates of noncompliance range from 8% to 95%. Korsch and Negrete (1972) did a study in which 53.4% of a group of mothers *satisfied* with their relationships with their pediatricians complied with instructions, while only 16.7% of the mothers who were *dissatisfied* with their relationship did so. Of the mothers who mentioned that they *liked* their physician's communication skills, 86% were satisfied. Only 25% of the patients who disliked the physician's communication skills were satisfied.

Noncompliance with prescribed medication regimens has been shown to be a significant cause of hospital admissions (Ley, 1988). Additional studies have revealed that patient compliance with prescribed medication falls to around 50% by the second visit to the physician and continues to fall to about 30% by the fifth visit (Phillips, 1988).

It has been reported that as many as 50% of patients leave a physician's office or clinic with little or no idea of what to do to care for themselves. They don't have even a rudimentary understanding of their medical problem, and they can't describe the treatment that is prescribed for them (Svarstad, 1976).

A recent study was designed to evaluate the relationship between the occurrence of malpractice lawsuits and the quality of communication between physicians and patients. The results clearly supported the hypothesis that physicians relating to patients in a negative manner (no eye contact, harsh and clipped tones of voice, criticism, minimal presentation of information and request for information, nonsmiling expressions, no friendly physical contact, no acknowledgment of verbalizations, no reflection of affect, no praise, and a relatively short contact) triggered increased litigious feelings when there was a bad result. However, physicians relating to a patient in a positive manner did not trigger such feelings. The authors explain that "the use of good communication behaviors, for example, may not be technically more 'competent' medicine, but it may prevent lawsuits, even when something has gone wrong and even when it is clearly the physician's fault" (Lester and Smith, 1993, p. 272). They conclude that physicians may be able to affect their risk of lawsuits by changing the way they relate to patients.

Another study identified the deficiencies of communication in the doctor-patient relationship that correlated with patient dissatisfaction and non-compliance as (1) poor transmission of information from patient to doctor, (2) low understandability of communications addressed to the patient, and (3) low levels of recall of information by the patient (Ley, 1988). In other studies, high levels of patient satisfaction were found to be related to (1) the physician's expression of warmth and courtesy toward patients, (2) the physician's empathic and encouraging questions eliciting patients' concerns and expectations, (3) clarifying and summarizing information received and conveying information at a level of discourse understandable to patients (Comstock et al., 1982; Korsch and Negrete, 1972).

TEACHING MEDICAL INTERVIEWING AND INTERPERSONAL SKILLS

Since the 1970s there has been a major surge in teaching medical interviewing and interpersonal skills. Some professional medical societies have become involved as strong advocates of interpersonal skill training, and some have developed their own programs for training physicians in the skills of interviewing and interpersonal communication. Among these societies are the following:

Association of Medical Colleges

Association for Behavioral Sciences in Medical Evaluation

Society of General Internal Medicine

Society of Teachers of Family Medicine

Task Force on Doctor and Patient of the Society of General Internal
Medicine

American Academy on Physician and Patient.

The last society includes teaching faculty from the specialties of internal medicine, family practice, ambulatory pediatrics, psychiatry, psychology, and other health care disciplines.

Virtually all medical schools now offer some teaching of medical interviewing and interpersonal skills. However, there is evidence that the quality of these programs varies considerably, "often providing students with uneven experiences and deficient skills" (Novak et al., 1993). Questionnaires were obtained from 114 deans and 92 course directors. They found that most schools encountered barriers such as lack of time, money, or resources. And faculty interest in teaching interpersonal skills had to compete with faculty support for traditional medical school courses. One study found that medical students' interpersonal skills with patients actually declined as their medical education progressed. The researcher concluded that in the medical training, the science of medicine replaces medicine's human dimension, with students finding it harder each year to talk with patients (Helfer, 1970). Another study found that the most important lesson learned by interns and residents is how to GROP (get rid of patients), and those who were good at it were called "dispo kids" (for disposing of patients). The researcher concluded that "the educational experience is structured to militate against the development of humanistic doctor–patient relationships" (Mizrahi, 1986, p. 119).

The pharmaceutical division of Miles, Inc., has developed a brief course of instruction in effective communication for physicians. However, because relationships between health professionals and patients require so many different skills, some of which can be learned only with extensive practice and coaching, the Miles course seems much too brief to bring physicians to a high level of competence.

BENEFITS TO BE DERIVED FROM EFFECTIVE INTERPERSONAL SKILLS

From our review of the research literature, we have compiled a surprisingly long list of tangible and concrete benefits to health professionals that studies have shown can be derived from effective interpersonal skills:

- Physicians gather more accurate data and make more correct diagnoses
- Nurses find out how patients are really feeling
- Patients have more trust in their caregiver

- Patient resistance to therapy and management will be reduced
- Patient catharsis and tension release are facilitated
- Negative nonverbal communication with patients is reduced
- Patient problem-solving promoted
- Health professionals are better equipped to counsel patients with problems in their lives
- Health professionals are more capable of helping patients cope in situations that exacerbate their disease
- Health professionals are more effective in dealing with specific groups of patients—difficult patients, aged or dying patients, the bereaved, adolescents, retarded and very young children, the chronically ill
- There is higher patient compliance with physicians' instructions
- There is greater patient satisfaction with visits to physicians
- There is higher assessment by patients of physicians' technical skills
- Patients are less likely to become helpless, dependent, and depressed when hospitalized
- Patients are discharged earlier from hospital
- Patients change physicians less often and are more likely to return to same practitioner
- Patients are less resistant to treatment
- Patients are less apt to bring malpractice suits
- Patients are less likely to seek out quacks and faith healers
- Patients are more likely to be optimistic and show a will to live.

Clearly, there is wide recognition of the benefits to be derived when patients are satisfied with their relationships with health professionals. It would seem that interpersonal communication skills training should be a critically important component of health care in this country. Many of the benefits listed above would significantly reduce the cost of health care— patients discharged earlier from hospitals, higher patient compliance, fewer malpractice suits, more correct diagnoses.

DIFFERENT CONCEPTS OF THE IDEAL
RELATIONSHIP WITH PATIENTS

Not only is there considerable awareness among health professionals that their relationships with patients have deteriorated, but surprisingly, the authors found in the medical literature frequent statements of what the relationship between health practitioners and patients ideally *should* be. We finally made a long list of the different ways the ideal relationship was described by health professionals:

- Person focus as opposed to problem focus
- Commitment to patients
- Humanistic professional as opposed to technological soldier
- Better bedside manner
- Style of the old family doctor
- Patient-centered as opposed to physician-centered
- More concern for patients
- Caring as well as curing
- More empathy with patients
- Treating patients with respect
- Fostering more patient involvement
- Compassion for patients
- Bonding with patients
- Unconditional, positive regard for patients
- Seeing patients as persons
- Listening more to patients
- Being a teacher to patients.

Although these terms and concepts are certainly very suggestive of what health professionals are perceiving as the critical elements in the "ideal" relationship with patients, they suffer from being far too nonspecific and abstract. They are terms that describe *attitudes*, *feelings*, and *values* rather than concrete and tangible behaviors. Scientists label such terms "nonoperational"—that is, they are both very difficult to put into operation and to teach.

TURNING ABSTRACTIONS INTO SPECIFIC BEHAVIORS

Hearing such nonoperational abstractions, it would be understandable if health professionals respond with:

What do I do to be empathic?

What do you mean by patient-centered?

How do I show caring for patients?

How do I get patients to participate?

Of course I see my patients as persons!

I have a lot of concern for my patients.

I certainly do a lot of listening with patients.

Imagine a tennis professional telling a student, "You need a more offensive backhand." Undoubtedly the student would agree and then say, "Well, how do I do that? Show me how I should grip the racket. How do I change my swing?" In training parents, too, it is essential to avoid such abstractions as "Give your child more love," "Treat kids with more respect," "See your child as a person," "Build a close relationship with your children," "Listen to your kids." Not only do such nonspecific representations make parents defensive, they don't tell parents what ineffective behaviors they are employing now or what behaviors would be more desirable.

Our review of the medical literature dealing with relationships with patients revealed too few descriptions of specific behaviors—either ineffective or effective. Our intention is to correct this oversight and share with the reader the specific interpersonal communication skills that can be used to greatly improve relationships with patients.

One of the principal objectives of this book is to make these abstractions more concrete, more operational, more usable. Abstractions will be reduced to specific behaviors, concrete actions, and proven skills that can be more easily understood, observed, illustrated, modeled, and taught. Building and maintaining mutually satisfying relationships with patients will require learning specific behaviors and skills, and also understanding when and when not to use them.

In simple terms, relating well to patients is much like learning to drive a car. There are many different skills for a driver to learn—steering, braking, accelerating, shifting gears, signaling, looking out for other cars, and so on. Learning to drive well, however, requires learning when and when not to use these skills, as well as when to use them simultaneously. So it is with learning the skills for developing mutually satisfying relationships.

Some communication skills are appropriate mostly for communicating empathy and acceptance of patients' behavior but are inappropriate, and consequently ineffective, for trying to influence patients to change their behavior. Certain communication skills are for sending *your* messages to patients, and different skills are used to encourage patients to send *their* messages to you. Some communication skills are appropriate for helping patients get *their* needs met, but other skills are called for when you are trying to get *your* needs met. For these reasons, building and maintaining good relationships with patients involves understanding and applying an integrated *system* of interdependent skills.

In the medical literature one can find articles that stress the complexities facing health professionals because they have to communicate with so many different kinds of patients. These articles allude to different styles of communication required for dealing with black or Hispanic patients as opposed to white patients, uneducated versus educated patients, male versus female patients, working-class patients versus those of a "higher social class" (Roter et al., 1988; Levy, 1985). The authors of these articles imply that health professionals need to adopt different communication styles for these different patient populations.

In this book, however, we will present a system of interpersonal skills that is generic to all kinds of patient populations. In fact, the reader will find these skills are equally applicable in all their interpersonal relationships— with their associates, their office staff, their spouses, their children.

The universality of these interpersonal skills greatly simplifies both teaching and learning them. It also means that health professionals won't have to assume different roles to match the different kinds of patients or people they deal with. Finally, it means that by utilizing the skills in all relationships, the reader will get a lot more practice, and thus become more proficient in a shorter period of time.

CHAPTER SUMMARY

In this chapter we provided evidence for widespread patient dissatisfaction in relationships with physicians and nurses. We cited examples of prominent health professionals calling attention to the need for humanizing relationships with patients, for "caring as well as curing." We cited evidence from a sample of research studies that patient dissatisfaction is associated with a number of poor patient health outcomes as well as with stronger litigious feelings. We called attention to the increase in the number of medical schools and medical societies offering training in medical interviewing and communication skills. We listed a large number of benefits to be derived from health professionals using effective communication skills and listed the different concepts and abstractions we found to describe the "ideal" relationship with patients. Finally, we emphasized the importance of identifying and teaching specific and operational behaviors and skills, as opposed to dealing with abstractions.

The next chapter will present a useful model for effective relationships between health professionals and patients—one that produces more active participation of patients in every phase of their relationship with health professionals.

Chapter 2

A Collaborative Model for Relating to Patients

Collaboration is a cooperative venture based on shared power and authority. It is nonhierarchical in nature. It assumes power based on a knowledge or expertise as opposed to power based on role or role function.
—William Kraus, *Collaboration in Organizations*

The evidence is very compelling that the way that many health professionals relate to patients could be significantly improved, and numerous research studies have identified an impressive list of specific benefits that would follow. The question to be asked now is whether there is an ideal or "best" way to relate to patients. What kind of relationship would be better than the traditional one, which has been shown to produce patient dissatisfaction and bring about poor patient health outcomes?

True, there has been growing agreement, particularly among medical and nursing educators, that training in interpersonal skills will increase both patient satisfaction and patient adherence to the prescribed medical regimen. However, there is not the same amount of agreement as to what kind of basic relationship with patients is needed. In this chapter we will make the case that health professionals are not likely to make use of interpersonal communication skills unless they first change their conception of the kind of relationship they want with patients.

For example, it has frequently been pointed out that physicians, and to some extent nurses, favor a relationship in which they are "in charge"—remaining in control of their interactions with patients. Anyone with experience in trying to teach interpersonal skills will recognize that in the conventional paternalistic model utilized in most relationships, there is little need for effective two-way communication. Parents and teachers unilaterally set the rules and expect youngsters to obey: "Do it because I say so." Authoritarian bosses also want to be in charge of almost every aspect of their relationships with subordinates, telling them what to do and when to do it, and tolerating no insubordination. In all those relationships, most communication not only is one-way, it is often dehumanizing and demeaning.

The same is true with the all too conventional relationship model so many physicians adopt. One of the physicians of the author (TG) asserted, "I'll do all the questioning." A famous heart surgeon is reported to have admitted that "most doctors don't want their patients to understand them because they prefer to keep their work a mystery. If patients don't understand what a doctor is talking about, they won't ask him questions. Then the doctor won't have to be bothered answering them" (Robinson, 1973). Such a physician-centered interviewing style has been said to dominate the delivery of most medical care in the United States today.

Nurses, too, seem to prefer a model of patient relationships that keeps them in charge. In one study it was found that a majority of the nurses and attendants on a geriatric ward reported changing the subject when patients tried to discuss their feelings about death. The most frequent reason they gave for doing this was that they wanted to "cheer up" the patient by focusing attention on something else (Kastenbaum and Aisenberg, 1972).

What is needed is a relationship model in which patients' communication is accepted and acknowledged—even welcomed. However, unless health professionals can be shown a model that they perceive will help them do their job more effectively and expeditiously, as well as build and maintain good relationships with their patients, they are not likely to want to make the effort to learn interpersonal communication skills. Even if they are taught these skills, they will not be motivated to use them unless they see the intrinsic value of a new relationship model—a new paradigm for their relationships with patients.

MODELS PROPOSED FOR RELATIONSHIPS WITH PATIENTS

A number of writers have advocated more collaboration and patient participation in the relationship between health professionals and patients. The authors of *Case Studies and Methods in Humanistic Medicine* write:

It is possible to expand these limited role definitions [caregiver is active, patient is passive], and the patient can learn to take a more active part in his care and to assume more responsibility for his health, *with the help* of the health professional. . . . By eliciting and using the patient's self-knowledge and inner resources, the practitioner can become more effective in the health care of his or her patient. (Belknap et al., 1975, p. 26)

Roter and Hall put it thus:

Most patients have a fear of committing social improprieties, doing the wrong thing, saying something stupid, being labelled a "bad" patient. This role prevents them from asking questions or requesting to see their medical charts. (Roter and Hall, 1992, p. 17)

Szasz and Hollander (1956) offer their own concept of an ideal relationship between health professionals and patients, a model that involves a contract in symbolic form. This model involves participation of patients in decision making, approximately equal power in the relationship, mutual interdependence, and activity that will in some way be mutually satisfying.

Stewart Miller, former director of the Institute of Humanistic Medicine, also argues for patients to be given a more active role, arguing that each patient has an "inner doctor" who at times can be mobilized in our own behalf, and become an active member of the health care team (S. Miller, 1975).

In assessing the character of physician–patient relationships, DiMatteo, a preeminent health psychologist, describes three basic models of the physician–patient relationship: (1) *the active–passive model*, where the patient is unable to participate in his or her own care; (2) *the guidance–co-operation model*, where the physician takes the bulk of responsibility for diagnosis and treatment; and (3) *the mutual participation model*, which involves physician and patient making joint decisions about every aspect of care, from the planning of diagnostic studies to the choice and implementation of treatment (DiMatteo, 1991). It is clear from the following that the author favors the third model:

There is joint input and joint responsibility. Typically, questions and concerns are aired freely. The mutual participation model represents the most effective physician-patient interchange that can occur. Physician and patient apply expertise to the task of achieving the patient's health. They can do this only with clear and effective communication. (DiMatteo, 1991, p. 194)

A similar but more complex system of classifying models of physician–patient relationships has been proposed by two Harvard physicians (Emanuel and Emanuel, 1992): (1) the *paternalistic model*, where the physician decides what intervention is best and tries to encourage the patient to consent; (2) the *informative model*, where the physician as the technical expert provides the relevant information and the patient selects the intervention he or she wants; (3) the *interpretive model*, where the physician provides information on both the medical condition and the risks and benefits of possible interventions. The physician also is a counselor, helping the patient through the process of deciding which values and course of action best fit the personality of the patient; and (4) the *deliberative model*, where the physician, acting as a teacher or friend, engages the patient in a dialogue to empower the patient to consider values and select a course of action that best fits his or her values.

The authors seem to favor the deliberative model, which they feel incorporates the aspects of caring for the patient while facilitating active participation of the patient in the entire process. They also admit that the deliberative model requires profound change in medical education and practice—such as teaching physicians to spend more time in physician–patient communication and developing a health care financing system "that properly reimburses—rather than penalizes—physicians for taking the time to discuss values with their patients" (Emanuel and Emanuel, 1992, p. 2226).

Allen B. Barbour, an internal medical specialist, describes a model of relationships between health professionals and patients as it would be in what he calls the "growth-model" of patient care, as opposed to the traditional "disease model":

We need to approach patients wholistically, if for no reason other than to practice a truly scientific medicine. . . . The patient and the health professional are colleagues. . . . The patient is encouraged to be aware of his choices and to become increasingly responsible for his own health, growth, and fulfillment. . . . We need to seek and apply ways to help our patients become more aware of their strengths and how to use them. Then, we can see ourselves as catalysts and as change agents—activating latent forces within our patients for their healing and growth. (Barbour, 1975, p. 50)

In an article titled "Partnerships in Patient Care: A Contractual Approach," Dr. Timothy Quill of the University of Rochester School of Medicine and Dentistry, strongly advocates a "partnership" with patients. Quill's model is based upon four concepts:

1. Each participant has unique responsibilities
2. The relationship is consensual, not obligatory
3. There is a willingness to negotiate
4. Each party must benefit from the relationship.

Quill further defines such a partnership:

He recommends that the patient must consider seriously, but need not follow, the recommendations made by the physician. If the patient and physician agree on a course of action together (that is, negotiate a contract), they become partners with well-defined obligations on both parts. . . . The patient may need to depend on the physician when sick, but need not always be submissive. The spirit of mutual participation expresses the willingness of doctor and patient to influence one another to govern the direction of treatment. (Quill, 1983, p. 229)

The value of a partnership between health professionals and their hospitalized patients was clearly spelled out by Dr. Ron Anderson, chairman of the board of the Texas Department of Health, in his interview in Bill Moyers's *Healing and the Mind.*

Well, in most hospitals we take your clothes away and give you a little gown with the back out of it. You may lose your dentures. Jewelry and other things that make you feel like a person are taken away. And you're supposed to be a good patient, therefore, you're obedient. Patients don't need to be obedient, they need to be able to complain, and to ask questions and to assert their point of view. You need to have a partnership, even though it can't be an equal partnership. We need to be the advocates for our patients in this partnership. That means they have to be empowered to complain without the fear that if they complained, they might lose their care. We want to empower them to learn how to take care of themselves when they go home, because they're going to be part of the health care team. Now not every patient can do this, but where you can, you develop a partnership with patients so that they can go home and understand the medication, for example. Or, if they have side effects, and you need to change the medication, then they become the ultimate decision-maker at home, and the doctor is the diagnostician, the person who initiated the therapy that was negotiated. (Moyers, 1993, p. 34)

In the literature we found these other terms for relationships with patients that were described and advocated:

Mutual problem-solving relationships

Patient-centered vs. physician-centered relationships

Open relationships

Two-way relationships

Mutually interdependent relationships.

BASIC ELEMENTS IN IDEAL RELATIONSHIPS WITH PATIENTS

In the ideal models that have been proposed, one can find some common basic elements that the advocates have judged desirable in relationships with patients:

Patients as active participants

Interdependence

Joint decision making

Empowerment of patients in their health

Two-way communication.

There are some other elements in these proposed models that don't seem realistic. Take the concept of the health professional and the patient as "colleagues." This concept overlooks the inevitable difference in expertise, experience, and medical knowledge in favor of the health professional. Similarly, the concept of "partners" could be misleading, inasmuch as that term so often implies an equal relationship, as in most business partnerships. However, the relationship with patients could be a partnership with each partner having unique expertise.

Several writers include the concept of "equal power" in the relationship. The problem with this concept is that neither health professionals nor their patients have *any* power—at least not the kind of power that parents have over their children, bosses have over their subordinates, and teachers have over their students. In fact, the relationship between health professional and patients is actually a consensual one, formed and existing by the consent of both. It is not an obligatory relationship, but its continuance does depend on both parties getting their needs met.

The idea that power is a component in relationships with patients is implied by writers who criticize health professionals for using their "authority," being "in charge," being "paternalistic," or being "authoritarian." These terms are as misleading as the concept of "equal power." We also found a model that contrasted "physician-centered" with "patient-centered." This same "either-or" thinking exists in adult–child relationships. Advocates of "power to the parent" and "dare-to-discipline" urge parents to assume an authoritarian role, and they defend that position by arguing that the only alternative is that the child will have the power to "rule the roost," leaving the adult with a passive and permissive role.

It's not commonly understood among parents, teachers, or managers that it is not necessary to make a choice between authoritarian (strict) and permissive (lenient) styles of leadership. There exists an alternative to being at either end of the strict–lenient scale—a third style. Does it fall in the middle of the scale—that is, moderately strict or moderately lenient? Not at all!

The alternative to the two either-or conceptions of human relationships, both of which are power based, is a model of relationships in which power isn't used at all! Such a relationship is not even on the power continuum— neither person is "in charge," neither tries to control, neither uses power. Such a nonpower, noncontrolling relationship has been called a cooperative relationship, a collaborative relationship, a synergistic relationship, an egalitarian relationship, a democratic relationship, or a partnership.

For this book the authors will use the term *collaborative relationship*, one that depends upon mutual participation and two-way communication. Collaborative relationships represent a paradigm entirely different from the kind of authoritarian relationships most of us have experienced—with our parents, teachers, and bosses. Consequently, we have incorrectly learned to expect that in all relationships one member invariably will have more power-based authority than the others.

To describe accurately the relationship between health professionals and patients, however, it is first necessary to recognize that there are multiple meanings of the word "authority." Unfortunately, we invariably use the same word to describe four different ideas.

Authority (Power)

Power-based authority—the capability to control, coerce, force, or compel others—is derived from possessing rewards or punishments. Rewards are the means to entice people to do something by promising some kind of benefit. "If you do this, I'll give you that." Getting the reward is contingent on doing what the controller wants. Punishments are the means to inflict pain or deprivation to get people to *stop* doing something, or to threaten pain or deprivation if they don't do it. People who use authority (power) are often called "authoritarians," but seldom do they use that term to describe themselves.

Authority (Expertise)

This kind of authority is derived from expertise, experience, or education. We employ consultants whom we think have this kind of authority. "He is an authority on infectious diseases." "She spoke with authority." People who possess this kind of authority are often said to be "authoritative" as opposed to authoritarian. This kind of authority is sometimes called "earned authority"—the kind that gives a person *influence* as opposed to *control*.

Authority (Job)

This kind of authority is based upon one's job description and the acceptance of others that in that job, one is expected and sanctioned to carry out certain specific duties, functions, and responsibilities. A police officer has the authority (the right) to direct traffic; an airline pilot has the authority to get passengers to fasten their seat belts; a hospital nurse has the authority to give baths or shots; a physician has the authority to write prescriptions. A person with this kind of authority is often said to be "authorized" to do certain things. Authority (job) gives people *influence* rather than *control*.

Authority (Contract)

This type of authority is derived from having made contracts, agreements, promises, or commitments with others. An author's contract with a book publisher gives the publisher the exclusive authority to print and sell the author's book. The author has been given the authority to receive royalties from the publisher. A patient agrees to have a physician perform an operation to remove a tumor. "I authorized him to do the surgery." "I agreed to stop taking my Coumadin three days prior to the surgery." Authority (contract) can strongly *influence* but does not *control* others.

Identifying these four different meanings of "authority" enables us to understand that in their relationships with patients, health professionals can safely utilize three kinds of authority: Authority (expertise), authority (job), and authority (contract). None of these involves control over others; they are all legitimate sources of *influencing* others. If health professionals attempt to use authority (power), which they don't actually have, it will alienate patients, and obviously it will rarely control the behavior of patients, except those whose learned reaction to authoritarians is to submit without question and resent it later.

THE CONSULTANT–CLIENT MODEL OF RELATIONSHIPS WITH PATIENTS

Having defined the different sources of authority, we can turn our attention to proposing a model for effective relationships with patients— one in which health professionals have these three sources of authority to influence their patients.

First of all, most people initiate a relationship with a health professional because they have evidence, or at least some hope, that he or she has expertise, experience, and knowledge. Physicians generally are perceived as having authority (expertise)—they are the expert *consultants* and have the credentials to prove it. Webster's Encyclopedic Unabridged Dictionary defines a consultant as "one who gives professional advice or services regarding matters in the field of his [or her] special knowledge or training."

Dr. C. Everett Koop also sees the physician as a consultant and has publicized his goal of training medical students to become "social consultants, humanitarians who value the art of medicine more than its financial rewards" (Koop, 1992). To accomplish this goal, the former surgeon general in 1992 joined the faculty of the Dartmouth Medical School, where he proposed that medical training should emphasize the importance of the doctor–patient relationship.

The model of physician as a consultant conforms to the fact that relationships with patients are consensual rather than obligatory. It also fits with the reality that health professionals generally find it necessary to give advice and to educate patients, much as consultants do. However, to be successful consultants, they need some additional skills, as we shall point out.

Successful consultants recognize the importance of withholding advice until they fully understand their clients' problems or their needs. Consequently, consultants are dependent on their clients to provide this critical information and thus need the appropriate communication skills to encourage clients' self-disclosure. Successful consultants recognize that their clients also possess some authority (expertise)—they have special knowledge of what is going on in their own organizations or in their lives. This makes the ideal consultant–client relationship a collaborative one—partnership between experts. As collaborators, each is important to the other; each has relevant data not available to the other; and they must develop effective two-way communication.

Unfortunately, few patients and few health professionals in their lifetimes have ever experienced a collaborative nonpower relationship. In fact, most of us have had authoritarian parents, teachers, and bosses who relied heavily on rewards and punishments to control our behavior. Consequently, many health professionals understandably lack the necessary skills to create and maintain a collaborative relationship involving influence rather than control. Similarly, most patients will perceive health professionals to be "in charge." They don't expect a collaborative relationship and wouldn't know how to act in one. Most important, because patients can't be expected to initiate or ask for a collaborative relationship, it has to be the health professional—the consultant—who must do it. However, health professionals first must be convinced of the benefits from, and the value of, fostering the active participation of patients in a collaborative relationship.

THE VALUE OF PATIENT PARTICIPATION

Ballard-Reisch proposes that there is value in participative decision making in the physician–patient relationship, in part because of the changing legal system that encourages patient knowledge and patient participation in medical decisions. Physicians may find that increased patient participation takes more time, yet in the traditional doctor–patient relationship, patients frequently misunderstand instructions, forget important procedures to follow in the treatment regimen, or fail to comply with their physician's instructions. Correcting such effects of inadequate or incomplete communication in the relationship frequently will require additional time later on (Ballard-Reisch, 1990).

Psychologists and other social scientists have been aware of the benefits of participation in relationships for a long time. Gordon Allport, one of the early giants in social psychology, summarized a number of experiments dealing with fostering participation in organizations and concluded that one "ceases to be reactive and contrary with respect to a desirable course of conduct only when he himself has had a voice in declaring that course of conduct to be desirable" (Allport, 1945). Bernie Siegel also has stressed the value of participation in "the healing partnership" between doctors and patients:

> Participation in the decision-making process, *more than any other factor*, determines the quality of the doctor–patient relationship. The exceptional patient wants to share responsibilities for life and treatment, and doctors who encourage that attitude can help all their patients heal faster. (Siegel, 1986, p. 51, italics added)

Siegel cites a research study at the University of Wisconsin Medical School in which Dr. Charlene Kavanaugh compared a group of severely burned children who received standard nursing care with another group who were taught to change their own dressings. Patients who had the more active role were found to need less medication and had fewer complications.

Other studies have shown the value of health professionals enlisting more participation and more input from patients and taking a less controlling and "in charge" role. One impressive study used the sophisticated statistical method of meta-analysis for combining the results of 41 independent studies. The findings showed a clear positive association between mutual participation through "partnership building," and both patients' satisfaction and their recall/understanding of their medical condition (Hall et al., 1988).

Dr. David S. Brody of the Temple University School of Medicine supports the view that increased participation of patients in clinical decision making would improve the quality and outcome of patient care for several reasons: (1) data collection would be improved, (2) the quality of clinical decisions would be enhanced, and (3) the physicians' use of technology would be combined with patients' concerns about the cost, inconvenience, discomfort, and dysfunction of medical interventions. In Brody's words:

> The act of incorporating the patient into the decision-making team tends to force the physician to consider all alternatives and explain the rationale behind the final recommendation. Armed with a basic understanding of the nature of the problem, the patient is now capable of constructively challenging the foundations of the physician's reasoning. This interchange should lead to a more rational, thorough, open consideration of the various alternatives. (Brody, 1980, p. 721)

Brody also sees significant advantages of patient participation, inasmuch as the traditional process of medical care often robs patients of control, self-reliance, and self-esteem, which can bring on dependency. Furthermore, patient noncompliance rates, which have been estimated from 25% to 50%, might decrease considerably as a result of patients having a stronger commitment to implement the treatment decisions in which they have participated.

In the field of organizational development the "participation principle," as it often has been called, is the critical element in a new kind of manager leadership—a style of supervising people that research studies have found brings about higher productivity, higher morale, fewer grievances, higher job satisfaction, lower turnover, and more willingness to comply with and implement solutions to problems.

In their pioneering book *Working Together*, John Simmons and William Mares summarize the findings from their study of 50 companies that use the participative management process for decision making and problem-solving:

> Productivity increases of 10 percent and more are not unusual and continue for several years. Early in the programs, productivity per employee may jump 100 percent. Grievances have fallen from 3,000 to 15, and stayed at that level. Absenteeism and turnover can be cut in half. . . . For some people who have led the way in introducing participation, the more important benefit has been human development. The material benefits are secondary. People feel better about themselves. They like to go to work. They have more self-esteem and self-confidence. They have gained control over their lives, if only a little, and lost some of their sense of powerlessness. (Simmons and Mares, 1983, p. 267)

The remarkable benefits of participation have also been proven in parent–child relationships. When given a voice in setting limits or rules they are expected to follow, children are more motivated to do so than when limits or rules are established by parents alone. Participation of children in rule setting also means less need for parents to enforce the rules and agreements. Enlisting children in setting family rules brings other benefits: decisions of higher quality, closer and warmer relationships between parents and children, more responsibility and self-discipline. And these children develop feelings of having control over their own destiny—what psychologists now call "fate control" (Gordon, 1976).

There are many occasions when health professionals and other caregivers can apply the participation principle to reduce patients' reactive and resistive behaviors. For example, a nurse given the responsibility for walking a patient every day might ask the patient, "Are you aware of any problems you might have carrying out the physician's orders to walk?" Or the nurse might ask what the patient would want to wear on his walks—slippers or shoes, pajamas or robe? Where would he like to walk? What time of day? How much physical support from the nurse? How far the first day? Would he want to increase the distance every day?

Hospice workers, too, will find the participation principle invaluable. The common tendency for terminally ill patients to become overdependent could be markedly reduced by giving them more opportunity to participate in making the many day-to-day decisions required in caring for such patients. Within this area of freedom, terminally ill patients could be encouraged to participate in choosing what foods they prefer, what hours they would like visitors to come, how they might relieve their loneliness at the hospice, when they prefer to go to sleep, and so on.

A corneal transplant patient shared with one of the authors a brief but intense conversation between herself and her surgeon during outpatient surgery in which she was encouraged to participate in solving a problem that helped her overcome strong anxiety feelings she had developed. The patient was to be given a local anesthetic and receive seven sutures in the left eye to adjust the curvature of the transplant. Before the surgery, while discussing options during an office appointment, the doctor gave her the following choice: (1) have sedation, which meant someone would have to drive her there and take her home afterward, or (2) not have sedation, so that she could drive herself to the outpatient surgery center and then drive home. She chose not to have sedation. She felt comfortable about her decision until soon after the procedure started, when she sensed there were a lot of people in the room. There were three surgeons observing her own surgeon, and she could hear everything they and the nurses were saying. Suddenly she felt terribly exposed, as if everyone were looking at her. She started experiencing anxiety, an overwhelming desire to jump off the table and run from the room. It began getting worse, but she hesitated to reveal to her doctor or the nurses that she was afraid and self-conscious. The anxiety was getting stronger by the second and she realized she was going to have to disclose her feelings somehow to relieve the stress. She knew that it was critical she not move during the procedure, so she tried talking it out:

Patient: I'm getting nervous.

Nurse: It's OK, Molly, you're doing fine.

[The patient said that she felt irritated when this nurse tried to deny her fears, reassuring her that she was doing fine when in fact she felt nearly out of control. The doctor, however, sensed the patient's urgency.]

Doctor: What's the matter, Mol? I'm right here.

Patient: I don't know. I'm getting nervous, and I want drugs.

Doctor: You can't have drugs, Molly. You wanted to drive yourself home.

Patient: I know, but I'm getting nervous and my stomach is empty and I'm hungry and I'm just feeling nervous.

Doctor: Well, what do you want me to do? Do you want me to talk? Do you want me to be quiet? What do you need?

Patient: Just talk me through each suture and tell me where you're at, so I know how close you are to being done.

Doctor: OK. We're doing great here. I'm almost done with the third one, and we've just got a few more to go.

The doctor continued guiding the patient through each suture until the end, as he agreed to do.

This patient reported that immediately after that conversation with her doctor, her anxiety completely dissipated; she felt comfortable and trusting almost instantly for the remaining 15 minutes in surgery. Because of this patient's ability and courage to self-disclose at a vulnerable and frightening moment, and her doctor's encouragement for her to participate in the proceedings, a potentially traumatic situation was resolved in a matter of seconds.

Dr. Peggy Manuel, a pediatrician who is an instructor of Parent Effectiveness Training (P.E.T.), shared with the author (TG) how she incorporated the participation principle with her child patients:

The P.E.T. course influenced me to discard using praise or ordering a child to sit still when I needed to do an ear examination. I adopted the practice of saying "I need to look into your ears," sometimes making it a game, like looking for Big Bird in the child's ear. Sometimes I let them look in my ears first or look in the parent's ears. A lot of times the child will say they really do see Big Bird in my ears. Mothers are usually very impressed, often telling me that this is the first time that the child did not cry when having the ear examination. I'm using the Principle of Participation, which may take a little longer but I find I don't have to struggle with children nearly as much. (Manuel, 1993)

In a speech to third-year medical students, patient Sandra McCollum spoke about the value of participation during the 50 times she was hospitalized with asthma/chronic bronchitis:

There are many concrete ways to include patients in their care. For example, my chart is available to me, whether I'm in the office or in a hospital bed. My doctor would routinely hold my chart so I can see lab results for myself, and if I can read his writing, I'm welcome to look at the notes or anything else in the record. I realize it isn't appropriate for you to allow all your patients to see their chart but can't you show them an X-ray or do something to include them in the process. . . . When you include us, when you give us choices about our care, you validate our lives and enable us to turn aside the pain and failure in even the worst situations.

The relationship we patients have with you, our physician, has a powerful impact on our lives. I'm very fortunate to have a variety of loving support systems. . . . You can tighten up the reins of control or let out the tether by trusting us. My physician authorizes refills on all my medications, including antibiotic prescriptions. He releases the reins of control by trusting me enough to know that I can usually tell when I need to begin antibiotics, and he knows I'll call him the next day if I do start taking the medicine. Recently, when he prescribed this inhaler (Ventolin), he asked me, "How many of these do you need to feel comfortable?" What an impact this had on me . . . I really need two inhalers—one in my nightstand and one in my purse—and to have all the bases covered, I like to have an extra in my desk drawer at work. In that brief question he healed a long-standing belief that I had an abnormal reliance on this crutch. (McCollum, 1992)

DEFINING COLLABORATIVE RELATIONSHIPS WITH PATIENTS

How can health professionals get their patients to participate actively in a collaborative relationship when most patients have never experienced such a relationship with physicians or nurses? Obviously, it's the health professional who needs to express his or her desire to have a collaborative relationship and then to define precisely what that means in terms of the roles each will assume. Following is an example of how a nurse might start out the relationship with a hospitalized patient:

Hello, Mrs. Elkins. Let me introduce myself. I'm Karen Hughes. I've worked here for four years now. My job is first to make sure the treatment regimen you and Dr. Blake agreed to gets implemented while you're in the hospital. Secondly, I'm here to hear what your needs might be and work with you to try and get them met. Then there are routine things that I or other nurses are required to do—take your temperature, do blood tests, give you your medicine [etc., etc.] .I want you to feel free to tell me whenever you have a problem or feel deprived or neglected. I'll do the same if something bothers me, as we work together to get you well.

This is only an illustration of how a nurse might begin a collaborative relationship with a patient. Exactly what is said would vary, of course, depending on the patient's illness and the hospital's procedures.

Here is an example of how a physician might express his or her preference for a collaborative partnership and describe what it would involve:

Mr. Clark, you've obviously come with some sort of concern or problem about your health. Let me explain that I much prefer working with each of my patients as a two-person collaborative team. This means we work together at all stages, beginning with defining your problem, deciding what will be needed to diagnose it, agreeing on the best diagnosis, coming up with a treatment plan, and evaluating how well the treatment worked. Think of it as a puzzle that we are going to work on together—trying to diagnose the problem as accurately as we can and agreeing on a treatment plan acceptable to both of us. It also means that we make sure we have open and honest communication between us, so if either of us is not satisfied during this process, we'll each communicate our problem to the other and then try to solve it. I'll want to take notes from time to time, and you should feel free to do the same. At any time feel free to ask questions.

Encouraging patients to ask questions is a very critical component of a collaborative relationship because most patients have been made to feel that they have relinquished the right to *ask* questions, yet they are all but required to *answer* almost any kind of question. Typically for most patients, asking questions is seen as the exclusive right of physicians, nurses, and other caregivers. One study revealed that more than half of patient talk in medical visits is giving information in response to the physician's questions. Only 6% of the 20-minute average visit is taken by patients asking the physician questions. Half the time of the medical visit, the physician is involved in doing things that don't even require the patient's presence (Roter and Hall, 1992).

Physicians also may need to make a special effort to emphasize that they want their patients to participate actively in the diagnosis phase of their relationship. In the typical relationship with patients, it's been the physician who assumes sole responsibility for making the diagnosis, and patients traditionally have accepted this.

The stereotype that diagnosis belongs in the doctor's job description has been challenged by clinical psychologist Dr. David Cain. He defines and evaluates three approaches to diagnosis:

Mechanical

Prescriptive

Collaborative.

In the *mechanical approach*, an expert is sought out by a person in need of assistance to determine the cause of the problem and to fix it. The car mechanic is a classic example of this model, but it also includes dentists, TV repairmen, and certain types of therapists, like hypnotists. In this model, the consumer derives no personal satisfaction or sense of accomplishment.

In the *prescriptive approach*, an expert makes a diagnosis of one's problem and prescribes a treatment. The physician is a prototype of this model. It also includes teachers, consultants, nutritionists, and physical trainers. The client (patient) later participates in the treatment or remediation. Nevertheless, the client's participation is usually passive, inasmuch as few practitioners involve their clients in developing a treatment regimen. The client is expected to comply with the expert's "prescription." The prescriptive approach requires little of clients with respect to their acquiring knowledge or skill, so the client remains dependent on the helper.

In the *collaborative approach* the client is an active participant in the diagnosis. Collaborative practitioners view their patients more holistically and are more person-focused than problem-focused. They have a goal of empowering their patients in an ongoing process of self-diagnosis. As a result, patients are more likely to feel satisfied through developing more "fate control" and less likely to feel dependent on the expert. The collaborative approach to the diagnosis process is another application of the participation principle. Here again, it must be the health professional who invites the patient to participate in this collaborative process and who communicates a description of just how they would relate as collaborators.

PARTICIPATIVE PROBLEM-SOLVING: THE SIX-STEP PROBLEM-SOLVING SYSTEM

The relationship between health professionals and their patients can be characterized as problem-centered in the same sense as a consultant–client relationship can be. Patients initially go to a physician because they have a health problem. In a collaborative relationship, physician and patient mutually participate to make decisions about what is causing the problem, what is concerning the patient, what among several alternatives should be the best treatment, what the patient must do to implement the treatment, how they will know if the treatment works, and so on. Indeed, all relationships involve problems to be solved. For example, husbands and wives are faced with all kinds of problems: Shall we have a baby? When? Shall we buy or rent? How should we invest our savings? Where should we go on vacation? Should we buy a new car? And so on ad infinitum.

It is widely understood by psychologists that relationships that are mutually satisfying and lasting are those in which the parties participate in solving their problems and end up with solutions that are satisfying to both. And their process is more likely to be effective and their solutions mutually satisfying when they employ a *system* of problem-solving—a blueprint they both can follow.

Such a system exists, and it has been shown to be effective. The author (TG) originally found it in the writings of John Dewey—as a system creative scientists often use for solving scientific problems. Later he applied the system to people problems—first to leaders in all kinds of organizations, then to parents, teachers, spouses, and others. Over a million persons have learned this problem-solving system. Consequently, we are confident that this system can be very useful to health professionals for solving the variety of problems that inevitably occur in their relationships with patients.

Called the *Six-Step Problem-Solving System*, it makes building and maintaining collaborative relationships easier. Without it, the parties often get hopelessly mired in unresolved conflicts, become angry antagonists, or terminate the relationship. Health professionals can easily learn the system; then they need to teach the system to their patients. A thorough explanation of each step is required. In fact, we recommend having the six steps displayed prominently in every consulting room.

As a device for illustrating this problem-solving system, we have created the following scenario showing how a physician might employ it during a patient's first office visit.

The reader is asked to approach this scenario by focusing primarily on the *process* rather than on the content. The content of such a clinical interview, of course, would be determined by the nature of the patient's medical problem and would vary a great deal with different kinds of problems. This scenario was written solely to illustrate how this model or system might apply to some theoretical patient's first visit.

It is also assumed that the physician in this scenario, Dr. A, would have already introduced herself and possibly would have asked the patient a few relevant open-ended questions, such as "How did you choose to come to me?" "How are you enjoying our sunny weather?" "Tell me about your work [or your family]," or whatever.

The physician (call her Dr. A) might set the stage by describing the collaborative approach briefly, why she prefers it, and its benefits. She might use such terms as "work together as a team," "both of us participating," "putting our heads together," "being partners," "assuming joint responsibility for solving your health problem," and so on. She may want to stress "two-way communication," "complete candor," "combining your personal experience with my professional experience," and so on. Then she might take the patient through each of the six steps of the system, perhaps using some kind of visual aid.

Step 1: Defining the Problem

Dr. A invites the patient to define her problem as she experiences it—her complaints, symptoms, feelings. She explains that her role will involve listening and perhaps some note-taking. Dr. A responds with empathic listening, asks for clarification when needed, keeps responsibility with the patient, avoids closed-ended probing questions, and encourages full patient disclosure. She may prime the pump with occasional open-ended questions, such as "Anything else you have experienced?" "Can you think of anything else that may be relevant?" "Anything more you want to tell me?"

When the patient is finished, Dr. A says she wants to do a physical exam and explains why. During the process she describes what she is doing, why she is doing it, and what she is finding. If she need not go further to make her diagnosis, Dr. A shares the diagnosis with the patient and invites reactions or questions.

If Dr. A thinks tests are needed to corroborate the initial diagnosis, she explains the nature of the tests and what the patient has to do to participate. After the test results are in (that same day or on some later day), she explains the results. If the diagnosis is that the patient has some specific disease, Dr. A describes the disease, verbally and/or with pictures or diagrams. She invites questions, reactions, and concerns. Dr. A listens attentively and with empathy, to show understanding and acceptance of the patient's feelings or concerns. She then may ask the patient to describe (feedback) the diagnosis to her in her own terms so she is certain the patient understands it.

Step 2: Generating Alternative Solutions

Dr. A now invites the patient's participation to generate possible solutions for correcting the medical problem as it was mutually defined in Step 1. She urges that neither should evaluate any of these alternative solutions until the list is complete. Depending on the diagnosis, several solutions might be generated from such alternatives as no treatment at all, certain medicines prescribed, more tests for further verification, referral to a specialist, surgery, obtaining a second opinion, complete rest and relaxation, a diet or exercise regimen, counseling, physical therapy, removing cause of stress, revision of personal habits, change in sleeping habits, reduction in working hours, and so on.

Step 3: Evaluating Alternative Solutions

When both feel they have exhausted all the alternative solutions generated in Step 2, Dr. A encourages the patient to participate with her in evaluating those alternative solutions (if there was more than one). What are the pros and cons of each? What are the costs? What are the risks? Are there time constraints? Is the best solution a combination of two alternatives? What are expected outcomes?

Step 4: Deciding on a Mutually Acceptable Solution

When all the facts are exposed and the alternative solutions weighed and analyzed, some best solution becomes clear to both physician and patient. Dr. A refrains from pushing a particular solution on the patient, recognizing that if the patient doesn't freely agree to the solution that best meets her needs, chances are the solution will not be willingly or completely implemented. She records the solution and checks with the patient as to the accuracy of the description.

Step 5: Implementing the Solution

Dr. A opens discussion about what now needs to be done to implement the solution. *Who* does *what* by *when* is useful framework for making a plan of action. Preferably, each person's tasks should be put in writing. The doctor agrees to carry out certain tasks—such as obtaining a date for admission to the hospital, authorizing X rays, writing prescriptions, and so on. The patient agrees to carry out certain tasks—getting prescriptions filled, going for X rays, taking the medication, using ice packs, checking her pulse—whatever.

Step 6: Evaluating the Effectiveness of the Solution

This final step is important but need not always be formalized. The patient may ask, "How will we know if our solution has solved the problem?" "How long do we have to wait?" "What do we do if the solution doesn't work?" "Are there tests to evaluate the effectiveness of our solution?" Dr. A acknowledges these concerns, of course, but the patient also deserves to be given Dr. A's best information about such things as the criteria for success or failure, the odds for success, what the patient might look for as evidence of its success, when relief might be experienced, and how soon. Dr. A urges the patient to write or phone her to inform her whether or not, or to what degree, their mutually determined treatment worked. They might agree on a date for a follow-up visit for this feedback.

THE BENEFITS OF THE SIX-STEP
PROBLEM-SOLVING METHOD

We have offered this simulation to illustrate how the Six-Step Problem-Solving Method could be utilized by physicians to facilitate patients' full participation in the problem-solving—including the diagnosis, treatment selection, treatment regimen, and follow-up.

Thirty years' experience teaching parents, teachers, and managers how to use the Six-Step System has shown that most people can quickly learn the process and obtain remarkable benefits. When people have been given the opportunity to participate in determining their destiny, they feel better about themselves, and have higher self-esteem, more self-confidence, and more fate control. They also feel they have been treated as an equal member of a team rather than as children or "second-class citizens." We have witnessed families, classrooms, and work groups quickly learn to function more collaboratively and, as a result, to have closer and warmer relationships than before. More often than not, participative problem-solving produces higher-quality solutions to problems—two heads are frequently more creative than one, because shared decisions are based on more data (Johnson et al., 1981). Finally, participative problem-solving produces higher motivation to implement the decision.

CHAPTER SUMMARY

In this chapter, we focused primarily on the overall relationship between health professionals and their patients—the traditional kind of relationship, new kinds of relationship models or paradigms that have been proposed, and common components of these models. We also attempted to clear up the semantic misunderstandings and problems with such terms as "power" and "authority." We introduced the notion that the ideal relationship between health professionals and patients might be likened to a successful consultant–client relationship, in which there must be active participation of both parties. We stressed the necessity for health professionals to assume the leadership in involving patients in this kind of partnership and pointed out the potential benefits of the participation principle.

Finally, we pointed out that people in all relationships must deal with problems and thus need to learn how to solve them effectively if those relationships are to endure. And we introduced a problem-solving system for strengthening and enriching relationships such as boss–subordinate, parent–child, teacher–student, and husband–wife. We proposed that this participative problem-solving system be used as a model by health professionals whenever they involve patients as participants to find mutually acceptable solutions to the various problems they encounter.

Chapter 3

Empathic Listening: Applications and Benefits

> It's a most terrifying feeling to realize that the doctor can't see the real you, that he can't understand what you feel and that he's just going ahead with his own ideas. I would start to feel that I was invisible or maybe not there at all.
>
> —R. D. Laing, *The Divided Self*

Health professionals who choose to adopt the collaborative consultant–client model for their relationships with patients will find it necessary to employ certain interpersonal communication skills that foster two-way communication, mutual problem-solving, and No-Lose Conflict Resolution. Such skills are seldom needed in typical relationships, in which one person is "in charge" and tries to control and dominate the other—such as most boss–subordinate, parent–child, or teacher–student relationships.

Experience tells us that very few persons have ever been in a truly collaborative, participative, or democratic relationship. Consequently, most people, including health professionals, haven't observed or been taught the critical communication skills needed to build and maintain truly democratic relationships. This chapter will identify and describe what we believe to be the most invaluable and indispensable of these unique interpersonal skills— empathic listening. We will first focus on the initial encounter between physicians and their patients, and later show how empathic listening can be used throughout the life of that relationship. We will also illustrate how nurses can utilize this useful skill in their relationships with patients.

THE INITIAL ENCOUNTER

There is something about one's first encounter with a new doctor, dressed in the white coat, that usually instills discomfort and fosters reticence. Most patients are already apprehensive, dreading the possibility of learning that they have something seriously wrong with them. Then there is the commonly experienced feeling of strong dependence upon this uniformed person you've just met. What will this doctor be like—friendly, overbearing, pressed for time, critical? Will I like this person? Will the doctor like me?

Physicians are also commonly perceived by patients as having greater "psychological size"—more education, more knowledge, more money, or belonging to a higher social class. The author (TG) has become aware of his practice of dressing up a bit more when he has a doctor's appointment. Then there are patients with medical problems that make them feel embarrassed to have to reveal or talk about them with another person, let alone get undressed and expose their less than perfect bodies.

All these feelings can be critical barriers to patients' open, honest, and direct communication with a new physician and, as a result, barriers to their active participation in this new relationship. How can these barriers be removed by physicians?

Patients will respond more positively to physicians who are cordial, friendly, relaxed, and unhurried. They will like physicians who are attentive to their physical comfort and perhaps engage in some brief small talk about unusual weather, the World Series game, important national news, bad traffic—whatever might be a timely or appropriate subject. Such questions as the following will convey the doctor's interest in you as a person, not just as a patient.

Tell me something about yourself.

How did you happen to choose to come to me?

If you have a job, what kind of work do you do?

Do you have a family?

Some physicians have long questionnaires to learn about their patients' health history. That same questionnaire could easily provide brief information about the patient's personal life—family members, sports activities, hobbies, travel, job, and so on. Or there might be a separate Personal Life Questionnaire. Not only would such information help physicians see the "whole person," but it would give them clues to what nonmedical subjects might be discussed at later visits with the patient.

Patients also bring to the physician's office many different thoughts about their particular health problem—expectations of the physician, concerns about what might cause their problem or how to communicate the difficult-to-describe symptoms they are experiencing, and the fears about the treatment to which they may have to submit. Any or all of these thoughts, if shared, could give the physician important clues and cues that would help define the problem accurately. Consequently, entering into the patient's unique perceptual self is the key for a physician to build a collaborative relationship—a joining of the patient's inner world with the physician's. What the physician must do to build such a relationship is exactly what successful consultants do—they use certain critical communication skills to get patients to start the interview, then they respond to what they hear by demonstrating their understanding and acceptance of their patient's messages.

BEGINNING THE CLINICAL INTERVIEW

After the brief initial encounter when small talk has been exchanged, the physician most frequently will have to be the one to speak first. (As an aside, the authors wish this procedure wasn't called an "interview," because the term implies that the physician's role is primarily one of asking questions of the interviewee, much as we see interviews conducted on TV. Nevertheless, "clinical interview" is the universally accepted term for physician and patient getting down to the business at hand—*defining the problem*, which is Step 1 in our Six-Step Problem-Solving Method, described in Chapter 2.

Although defining the patient's medical problem may be the primary goal of the clinical interview, we would strongly urge physicians to keep in mind additional functions or goals of the interview: (1) demonstrating their empathy, (2) confirming their understanding and acceptance of patients' communications, (3) reducing their "psychological size," and (4) enlisting full participation of the patient in this collaborative relationship. It has been pointed out repeatedly in the literature that programs for training medical students usually assume that the chief or sole purpose of the clinical interview is "history taking," with insufficient emphasis on building rapport and fostering a relationship (Bird and Cohen-Cole, 1990).

The additional functions we suggest for the clinical interview are those that would serve to establish a collaborative and participative relationship with patients. To this end it would seem logical that physicians invite patients to begin the procedure by describing their medical problem in their own words.

With the patient starting the procedure, the physician then has the opportunity to use the skills that will *demonstrate* being empathic, understanding, and accepting. This will encourage the patient to give full information, define the basic problems and needs, and begin to feel that his or her active participation in this relationship is encouraged. We will first focus on the potent listening skill the physician will need, particularly in the early stages of the procedure. Later, naturally, the physician will need to do more than listen when it seems appropriate to add his or her inputs to those of the patient.

THE CRITICAL LISTENING SKILL

Because it is the patient who made the decision to see the doctor, the patient should be invited by the doctor to begin:

Tell me what brought you here today.

Where do you want to start?

I'd like you to describe your problem.

In your own words, tell me about your health problem.

Attending Behaviors

Attending behaviors are essentially physical postures that convey the physician's desire to get involved with, show interest in, and focus almost exclusively on what the patient is communicating. Attending is also one way of demonstrating caring. One writer has described proper attending as "relaxed alertness." It usually involves the caregiver in a physical position of inclining his or her body toward the speaker, facing the person squarely at eye level, and taking a position at an appropriate distance from the patient. Being too distant may block communication; sitting or standing too close may cause discomfort. Some trainers of professional counselors suggest the distance of around a yard. Skilled listeners typically nod or shake their head when touched deeply. Probably the most critical component of attending is consistent eye contact, avoiding glances around the room or at your watch and avoiding keeping your eyes glued on your paper when taking notes. Physicians who at first feel uncomfortable with intense eye contact may begin by focusing on the speaker's mouth—later on the eyes.

Understandably, physicians may wonder, How can I take notes during the interview with patients if I'm supposed to keep looking at them when they're describing their problem or health history? While that is a common question, there are some possible solutions. They might consider audiotaping the initial interview. Or when they feel a need to make a note on something important the patient has said, they might say, "Would you mind stopping for a moment to let me make a note of what you just reported?"

Positioning yourself on one side of a desk between you and the patient may seriously inhibit open and honest patient self-disclosure. Desks usually symbolize a position of authority and can promote dependency or fear of judgment. Some physicians have reported placing a chair to the side of a desk or coming out from behind their desk.

Physically attending is more important than people think. Experts in the field of communication report that as much as three-fourths of person-to-person communication is nonverbal. So if physicians keep their attention on patients, it will contribute greatly to the patients' perceiving that their talk is wanted, that the physicians are really trying to understand what they're communicating, and that they care.

Passive Listening

Saying nothing is a potent skill that professional consultants use extensively with their clients. Passive Listening can provide patients with time to think what they're going to say next, and it often encourages them to move from a "presenting problem" to a more basic problem. However, silence does have the limitation of not giving adequate proof to patients that they have been accurately understood.

Passive Listening can be made somewhat more interactive by inserting simple, noncommittal acknowledgments such as "I see," "Uh-huh," "Oh." If it seems appropriate, one can offer encouragers such as "I sure understand that," "I hear what you're saying," "Yeah," "Interesting," or "How about that?"

Even with such brief acknowledgments, Passive Listening does not definitely *prove* to senders that their message has been accurately understood and truly accepted. In fact, silence to some patients may suggest that you're "not with them" because they think you're daydreaming about something in your own life instead of understanding what they're saying. Fortunately, there is another kind of listening that does not have these limitations or risks.

Active Listening

Counselors and psychotherapists in the 1940s discovered a new kind of listening that strongly encourages a person's *self-disclosure,* demonstrates *empathy*, proves *accurate understanding* of what is disclosed, and conveys *acceptance* of what was heard (Rogers, 1951).

One of the consistent findings, from both research and the experiences of the counselors, was that self-disclosure of the counselees was greatly facilitated by a response that was first called the counselor's "reflection of feelings." Later the term "Active Listening" was used in Effectiveness Training courses, and it became almost universally accepted for this empathic way of responding to others.

Active Listening, viewed simply as a verbal skill of responding to another person's communication, is rather easy to describe. It involves listening attentively, then "feeding back" to the sender your understanding of the meaning of the sender's message. This can be represented by a series of diagrams. It begins with a SENDER experiencing something inside—a feeling, a need, a fear, an attitude, or an idea. For example, let's have a patient as the SENDER feeling worried. Her physician will be the RECEIVER.

Because it is not possible for the worried patient to describe all the complex physiological and mental processes actually going on inside her organism, she must select some words that she thinks might represent to the physician what is going on inside. This selection process is called "encoding"—choosing some sort of a code to carry a message to the RECEIVER. Let's say this patient selects the words (the code) "I can't stop thinking it's going to be cancer." Now the RECEIVER, wanting to understand the SENDER, has to "decode" the message, a mental process that is a form of "translating" the code. However, because one can never be sure exactly what is in another's mind or body, the RECEIVER'S decoding process usually involves making an educated guess: "I think she is really worried."

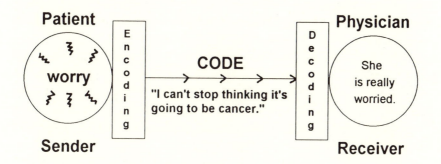

However, not feeling completely sure of the accuracy of his decoding, the physician checks it out by sending the decoded message back to the patient. He obviously refrains from sending some new message, one that communicates what *he* is thinking, such as "I'm pretty sure it isn't cancer." Instead, he "mirrors back" *only* what he thought was in the patient's mind. This response is called a feedback:

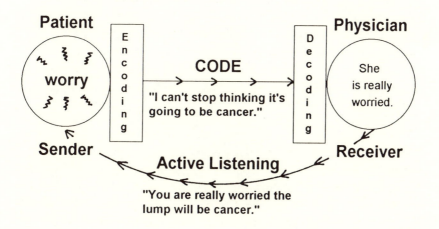

Now the patient can either confirm the accuracy of the feedback, modify it, or reject it. In this case, the patient probably would confirm by saying, "Yeah, I am very worried," thus telling the physician that he had put himself in her shoes (was empathic), had accurately understood her message, and had accepted her feeling worried.

Diagrams, however, do not adequately describe the essence of Active Listening. First, it requires the listener to put aside his or her own thoughts and feelings for a moment, shutting out as completely as possible his or her way of looking at things, in order to understand the speaker's personal and unique thoughts or feelings—what psychologists call a person's "phenomenological self." Active Listening requires the listener to empathize with the speaker, momentarily to identify with the speaker, enter into the world of the speaker's view of reality. Active Listening is *the* skill par excellence for communicating "understanding" and "empathy"—those two abstract terms that are found so frequently in articles and books that describe an ideal relationship between health professionals and their patients. While it seems to be almost a consensus that health professionals *should* be understanding and empathic toward patients, seldom are they told precisely how to do that. Empathy is generally understood as identifying with or experiencing the feelings or thoughts of another person. But how does a person show that? How does a person *prove* to the speaker that he or she has understood? Active Listening is the answer to those questions.

Robert Bolton, author of *People Skills*, quotes from Milton Mayeroff's book *On Caring*, in which the latter identified the components of empathy and caring:

> To care for another person, I must be able to understand him and his world as if I were inside it. I must be able to see, as it were, with his eyes what his world is like to him and how he sees himself. Instead of merely looking at him in a detached way from outside, as if he were a specimen, I must be able to be with him in his world, "going" into his world in order to sense from "inside" what life is like for him. (Bolton, 1979, p. 272)

Although empathy is momentarily experiencing another person's way of seeing the world, the listener of course does not lose his or her identity. Also, empathy is *feeling with* another, not at all like sympathy, which is *feeling for* another. Empathizing with another can be facilitated by asking oneself, "If I were having the same experience as the sender, what would be my feelings, thoughts, or reactions?" "What does it feel like to the sender?" "What is in the sender's awareness at this moment?"

Active Listening has also been described as a *receiving* of another's experience rather than a *projection* of one's own feelings onto the other person. A nurse, speaking of empathy, once said, "I have the opportunity to experience a thousand different lifetimes through someone else's eyes."

In her article "Caring vs. Curing," Carol Montgomery links Active Listening with caring, another abstraction we found so often in the literature. She describes the findings from her interviews with 35 nurses referred to her as exemplars of caring:

> What emerged as an overriding element of caring was spiritual tran-
> scendence—i.e. in opening herself to a relationship with another, the
> caregiver experienced herself as part of a force greater than herself.
> This finding challenges the conventional assumption that one must
> maintain distance and objectivity to be an effective helper. . . . This
> approach in helping is very different from the achievement-oriented
> one that aims to cure disease and eliminate problems. While these
> goals appropriately represent one aspect of what nurses—and thera-
> pists—do, they need to be distinguished from the caring aspect. When
> our agenda is to fix or cure, the focus is on ourselves as "ego-heroes."
> (Montgomery, 1991, p. 38)

Paraphrasing one of the nurses in her study, Montgomery writes: When we allow someone to become part of our hearts, helping to heal that person heals our hearts as well.

The critical importance and effectiveness of Active Listening for expressing empathy and facilitating patient self-disclosure is clearly understood by Paul Bellet and Michael Maloney at the University of Cincinnati College of Medicine:

> The use of empathy as an interviewing skill involves learning to
> understand patients in depth. The interview is potentially the most
> powerful, sensitive, and versatile instrument at the physician's com-
> mand. . . . The physician should ask open-ended questions and reflect
> back to the patient the way the patient seems to be feeling. . . . A test
> of one's empathic accuracy is the extent to which the physician's
> responses stimulate and deepen the patient's narrative flow. . . . The
> feeling of being understood strengthens the working alliance between
> the patient and physician. An important factor in accepting a physi-

cian's advice is the patient's perception of the physician's empathy for the illness and related concerns. (Bellet and Maloney, 1991, p. 1831)

Empathic caring is only one of the necessary elements of the Active Listening process. A second component is checking on the accuracy of the listener's *cognitive understanding* of the message. Because we can never be certain that we have accurately understood what another person is experiencing and trying to communicate to us, we make an effort to find out. When using Active Listening, the receiver doesn't remain silent after hearing what is communicated but puts what he or she has understood *into his or her own words* (code) and then feeds its back to the sender to get verification, modification, or correction. This is the interpersonal communication skill for providing evidence to both the receiver and the sender on whether accurate communication has been achieved. And what a time-saver that can be in relationships!

Another obvious benefit of Active Listening in the medical interview is to give the physician a way to elicit from the patient the maximum amount of relevant information. Here are two example dialogues submitted by Dr. Ralph Riffenburgh, a physician in one of the author's earliest training groups (Riffenburgh, 1974). In the beginning of the first dialogue, the physician did not use Active Listening until he became aware of the patient's resistance to his probing questions:

Example 1

A physician is seeing for the first time a 47-year-old man with intermittent upper abdominal pain. The occurrence of the pain, which is somewhat suggestive of ulcer, may be related to difficulties on the job.

Patient: But I had the last attack when everything was going well at work. Old Mr. Driver retired several months before—he always made confusion—and the work wasn't particularly heavy. I wasn't staying late that month at all.

Doctor: Did Mr. Driver's retirement throw more responsibility on you?

Patient: No. He didn't really do his work right and when Jim took his job, I could count on the people who handled the invoices before me doing them correctly—Jim has really shaped those slobs up. My wife felt I should have had Driver's job but I couldn't do nearly as well as Jim.

Doctor: Does your wife push you to get promoted?

Patient: No.

[In this monosyllabic answer, the patient shows resistance, so the doctor stops his probing questioning and starts to feedback with Active Listening.]

Doctor: You do like working for Jim?

Patient: He is a remarkable leader and does a fine job. That position would frighten me, as I don't do so well controlling others.

Doctor: So not getting that promotion was OK with you? (ACTIVE LISTENING)

Patient: I really didn't consider it. When Mr. Jackson retires or moves up, I would like his job. It is the same level as Jim's but requires control of figures and financial planning rather than making other people perform. I realize that this is my strong point rather than dealing with people.

Doctor: Then you are willing to wait for a promotion to get the type of job you are good at and you would enjoy. (ACTIVE LISTEN-ING)

Patient: That's right. I feel I understand my limitations. My wife can't understand this, as the two jobs are at the same level.

Doctor: Your wife doesn't understand the difference in the requirements of the two jobs? (ACTIVE LISTENING)

Patient: No, she doesn't, and it really bothers her that I have been with the company longer than Jim has. She really put the pressure on me when Jim and his wife bought their new house in the Heights—she has wanted to move and we can't afford it on my salary.

Doctor: So Jim's move really got to her. (ACTIVE LISTENING)

Patient: Oh, yes. Jim had an open house for the department in his new house, and she was furious when we got home. Come to think of it, the attack started that week.

Doctor: So pressure for promotion may be a factor, as well as when things are bad at work. (ACTIVE LISTENING)

Patient: It sure looks that way. I wish she could understand how I feel about the type of work I do well.

Doctor: Does the pain seem to be better or worse after you eat?

[Having brought the issue of promotion pressure out in the open, the doctor now returns to the standard questioning techniques of the medical interview in order to get more diagnostic detail about the symptoms. The patient is now able to recognize the impact of his wife's resentment and the doctor might well return to the subject in discussing means of coping with the symptoms.] (p. 93)

Example 2

A physician has completed interviewing and examining a patient with recurrent headaches.

Doctor: I think you are suffering from migraine headaches.

Patient: But I get sick to my stomach with them.

[The doctor explains the mechanisms of nausea in migraine.]

Patient: Painkillers don't seem to help.

[The physician realizes that something else is on the patient's mind, blocking her acceptance of his diagnosis. Instead of further explanations, he tries to bring out her underlying apprehension.]

Doctor: The headache worries you as well as giving you pain. (ACTIVE LISTENING)

Patient: I wonder what the real cause is.

Doctor: You feel that there is something behind the headache which we haven't found? (ACTIVE LISTENING)

Patient: In some ways it sounds like the headaches that my aunt had.

Doctor: And you don't like the idea of having the type that she had? (ACTIVE LISTENING)

Patient: Months of treatment didn't help her at all.

Doctor: She had something more serious than the doctors suspected? (ACTIVE LISTENING)

Patient: She died of a brain tumor.

[Now the underlying cause of the patient's fear is out in the open.]

Doctor: Brain tumor is one of the first things we considered in your case, and I'm sure that you do not have that. Your headaches fit a well-established pattern and should respond to treatment. Now I want to explain the mechanism of some of your symptoms.

[Now the patient is able to listen and understand the explanations. Her underlying fear had been so dominant before the possibility of brain tumor was first mentioned and refuted that she didn't really listen to the doctor's diagnosis or explanation.] (p. 93)

Dr. Robert Daigneault, a physician trained and authorized as an Effectiveness Training instructor, contributed this account of his using Active Listening with a graduate student:

The following exchange occurred when a 28-year-old graduate student came to my office with a complaint of tiredness of several months' duration. He found that he was having problems with his studies and did not want to fail. I initially proceeded in the standard manner by taking a history and doing a physical exam. I also ran a few lab tests and had him return for discussion of the lab results. At his next visit I began by telling him that the workup so far was negative and therefore the tiredness was probably not physical in nature.

Graduate Student (GS): I really don't think this is an emotional problem, Doc. I mean, I'm just tired.

Dr. D: You don't believe an emotional problem could make you this tired. (ACTIVE LISTENING)

GS: Right. It must be something else, because everything's OK at home.

Dr. D: You don't feel that there are any problems at home. (ACTIVE LISTENING)

GS: No. I mean, my wife and I occasionally argue about my program and money. It bugs me.

Dr. D: Arguing with your wife upsets you and makes you feel bad. (ACTIVE LISTENING)

GS: Yes, I mean I'm trying. I'm just feeling too tired to do things.

Dr. D: You're annoyed with your wife because she doesn't understand that you're trying to do your best. (ACTIVE LISTENING)

GS: (nods in agreement) These arguments are really getting me down. I hate going home. Life's no fun anymore.

The dialogue continued and it became clear that GS was depressed. I treated him briefly with anti-depressants and saw him for a few counseling sessions. He was able to finish his program and went on to a teaching career.

FREQUENTLY EXPRESSED CONCERNS ABOUT
ACTIVE LISTENING

Because the Active Listening skill is new to most people, it invariably provokes some concerns and raises some questions.

Will Using Active Listening Be Time-Consuming?

One of the most frequent concerns of physicians using Active Listening is that it will take too much time. Physicians already are working under severe time pressures, so it's understandable they would be concerned that this skill would encourage patients to talk more—to bring up new feelings and needs, invite lengthy catharsis.

Some medical writers defend empathic listening as likely to *save* time, as well as expense, as in the following excerpt:

. . . . Physicians in clinical practice may feel that they do not have enough time for empathy. In the long run, though, empathy may save much time and expense. Without a sense that his or her physician is empathic, a patient feels alone and alienated. With it [empathy], the patient feels that the physician understands. This may decrease anxiety, so that the patient is more amenable to accepting the physician's advice. (Bellet and Maloney, 1991, p. 1832)

The long-range outcomes from empathic listening were listed in a journal article that advocated physicians taking the time to listen:

When one begins to listen to patients several things happen. Major, as opposed to initial, complaints are clarified and addressed. The personal style of the patient becomes clear, so individualized treatment may be used with enhanced [patient] comprehensiveness and compliance. Psychological and social complaints and maladjustments are put into proper context in the care process. (Lipkin et al., 1984, p. 277)

In a speech to physicians, a knowledgeable and insightful asthmatic patient had this to say about physicians taking the time to listen to their patients:

I suspect at this point some of you must be thinking, "This is all well and good, but who has the time to develop this kind of rapport?" None of us ever has enough time. But think about how much time you will spend over the year practicing defensive medicine—the minutes you spend considering whether to order that test or that procedure—just in case this is the person who will haunt you five years later with a subpoena. Investing in a trusting relationship is the best defense against a lawsuit. (McCollum, 1992)

In a study conducted in South Africa, the researchers found that the frequent assumption that it takes longer to conduct a patient-centered consultation was *not* supported by their findings: "Lack of time cannot be legitimately offered as an excuse for not conducting patient-centered consultations" (Henbest and Fehrsen, 1992, p. 316).

Won't Active Listening Sound Like Parroting?

We have encountered resistance to Active Listening based upon the impression that those who use the skill will sound like parrots, which will seem ridiculous to patients. Naturally, parroting back their messages in their identical words would put off most patients. An effective Active Listening response should be in the listener's own words, indicating that the listener has accurately decoded the message and understood its meaning. Parroting the patient's code rarely proves understanding of the patient's inner feelings. *Remember: the code is not the message.*

Is Active Listening Too Difficult to Learn?

When first introduced to this important skill, people do tend to think it is so new and different from the way they are used to responding to others that it will be very difficult to do it effectively. Although it does require consistent practice, there is a built-in feature of Active Listening that facilitates learning to be competent at it—namely, the sender's response to the listener's feedback. If the feedback is an accurate one and carries the same degree of feeling as the message, the sender will usually verify this—first by saying, "That's right," "Yeah," "It sure did," or some other confirming response. On the other hand, if the listener's feedback is inaccurate or doesn't carry the feeling in the sender's message, the sender will typically say so with such responses as "No, that's not it," "I don't mean that," "Not exactly," "You don't understand." And, being even more helpful to the listener, the sender who feels misunderstood almost invariably will send a second message, somewhat differently encoded from the first, giving the listener another chance.

This common corrective response to an inaccurate feedback is precisely what accelerates becoming proficient with Active Listening—an excellent validation of "practice makes perfect."

Feeding Back Without Empathy

Not every message sent by patients carries feelings, but most do. Patients also send solely cognitive or informational messages carrying no feeling—such as "The pain is always in my right shoulder" or "I have trouble sleeping at night." Such clearly coded messages don't require feedback. However, when the message does contain feeling, it's important to acknowledge it with Active Listening. We all respond favorably when someone understands how we feel, as well as just the factual content. Patients particularly send lots of messages that contain such feelings as fear, disappointment, frustration, worry, helplessness, sadness, and so on. If physicians fail to feedback such feelings, patients naturally will feel that the essential part of them at that moment is not being understood.

In our Effectiveness Training courses, we find some people who are very uncomfortable with feelings—they want to push feelings out of the picture, hide them, deny them. However, when they make the effort to hear others' feelings and empathize with them, they learn that feelings are often transitory—especially if they are acknowledged and understood. More often than not, feelings are friendly—they can be very informative and lead to new understandings in relationships.

OTHER APPLICATIONS OF ACTIVE LISTENING

We have so far presented Active Listening as an indispensable skill for physicians to employ in the initial clinical interview. By no means is this the only time it's useful. In fact, this method of communicating empathy, understanding, and acceptance has such general usefulness that it might be called the all-purpose skill. Its versatility has been proven in a wide variety of situations.

Active Listening is a critical skill for nurses and other caregivers to build good relationships with patients. It can be effectively utilized when patients develop strong feelings—such as dissatisfaction with what they are asked to do, concerns about being away so long from family members, upset with receiving a lot of shots or giving so many blood samples, distress over an unfavorable diagnosis of their medical problem, irritation over the food they have to eat, doubt about the physician's treatment recommendation, dissatisfaction with how infrequently their doctor visits them, and so on. When patients express such feelings, nurses and other caregivers have the opportunity to show their empathic understanding by avoiding the 12 Roadblocks and using Active Listening.

Messages patients send when they are experiencing problems may be either verbal or nonverbal. Nonverbal messages often are unclear, indirect, and so highly coded that the receiver will have difficulty trying to decode them. Seldom are patients—or anyone else, for that matter—consistently open, honest, and direct in revealing their problems to another. But they do give off nonverbal clues. Here is a small sample of patients' nonverbal clues:

Becoming suddenly quiet, noncommunicative

Changing facial expression

Looking away or down

Getting fidgety, shaky

Making some hand gesture

Looking sad, downcast

Not eating anything on their tray.

Health professionals should not ignore such nonverbal clues, but instead respond with a tentative Active Listening response to show acceptance and invite more self-disclosure, which, one hopes, will be a verbal communication that gives more information:

You seem upset (or sad or worried, etc.). Am I right?

Do I detect that you have a concern about my fee?

Something on your mind?

Do you want to tell me something?

You don't seem yourself today.

Anything wrong?

Here are examples of verbal messages patients might send that are coded rather unclearly—they are not clear and direct:

Not another X ray?

(To nurse) Wish I could be as cheerful as you are.

(To nurse) When do I get out of this jail?

It's all Greek to me.

(To nurse) Do I have to get on this damn scale again?

What have I done to deserve this?

Are you telling me all I should know?

To respond to both nonverbal and unclearly coded messages, health professionals will have to do some fancy guesswork—what we call speculative decoding. Then if the feedback is not correct, the patient will undoubtedly send a second message with a different (and, one hopes, a clearer) code. However, should the health professional make a shrewd guess and send an accurate feedback, the patient generally will confirm the accuracy of the feedback with "That's right," "I'd say so," "That's what I feel," "Right." Or the patient will go deeper into a more basic problem.

Active Listening is what really completes an accurate communication process, thus eliminating a lot of misunderstandings between persons. Of course, it often takes more than one such feedback to produce complete understanding, as in this dialogue:

Patient: How confident are you about your diagnosis?

Doctor: You're worried that I might be wrong?

Patient: No. I was *hoping* you might be wrong!

Doctor: You hate hearing my diagnosis of stomach ulcer, right?

Patient: Yeah. It means going on a lousy bland diet with no liquor at all!

Doctor: You're afraid it will be hard for you to give up drinking.

Patient: Terribly hard!

Obviously, patients sometimes will come right to the point and encode so clearly and concise that the meaning is very clear:

Nurse, it's hard for me to get a good night's sleep with the door open. Could it be closed?

Such a clear message doesn't always need a feedback. If the nurse answers the request with "Sure, I'll close it when I leave," it's obvious to the patient she has understood the message and solved the patient's problem.

Using effective Active Listening, physicians may find out that they are part of the patient's problem, and thus may be the only one who can provide the solution by giving information or changing their behavior. Rarely do people come right out and with only one message clearly reveal the real or basic problem they are having. They usually begin by sending an indirect message about something else—what counseling professionals call the Presenting Problem. Here are some examples of such messages:

I hope I'm not sounding like a hypochondriac.

Could this be caused by stress?

How much is too much alcohol?

I'm too young to have a hysterectomy.

Often such messages will lead to a more basic problem, thus providing the health professional with more critical information. Active Listening has the remarkable ability to facilitate the sender's going deeper and deeper, until he or she can verbalize the basic problem. This may take a minute or it may take much longer. Here is an example of a patient with multiple complaints, on 9 medications and averaging 20 medical visits per year. She began by telling her physician about a presenting problem of being constantly fatigued. In the words of the physician:

We talked for quite awhile, until she gradually acknowledged the many hardships that were the reality of her life. She sensed the affirmation and caring that were part of my attentive listening, and she was encouraged to continue. In the course of a half-hour's recital, she gradually came into a clear awareness of the tremendous stresses of her life and, equally important, she saw for the first time her own inner strength in being able and willing to cope with those stresses over the years. My own interventions were simply restricted to affirming, from time to time, the truth of what she was seeing in such detail—the truth of her life. Through this process of sharing the facts and predicaments of her life, she emerged from the interview with a great deal more confidence in herself. She also gained confidence in me as her physician as a result of my accepting who she was, complete with problems and turmoil. I was pleased and impressed that she was able to see the absurdity, as well as the tragedy, of her situation after this visit. After a few more such visits she wanted to reduce her medications and to limit her medical visits to two each year. I concurred with her in these decisions. (Belknap et al., 1975, p. 28)

The following dialogue was submitted by a patient who strongly resisted her doctor's treatment solution:

Patient: I hear your strong recommendation that I should have a hysterectomy, but I don't have any symptoms that are interfering with my life. I'm not ready to have that surgery.

Physician: Since you're not having problems, you don't want surgery now.

Patient: That's right. What I'd like to do is consider other alternatives.

Physician: You'd like to see if there might be some other way to treat the fibroids.

Patient: Yes, that's right. Do you know something else I might try?

Physician: No. No one has ever asked me about this before. I do know a doctor here who might have some experience with holistic treatments for women with fibroids. Why don't I do some research on this and call you in a couple of weeks?

Patient: Great! I would really appreciate that.

Physician: I'd like to work with you on this.

The patient reported that she really felt accepted by her gynecologist and supported by her willingness to help her.

Here is another example of using Active Listening to help a patient disclose his fear of spinal anesthesia, which led to his finding a unique solution to that problem. The patient is talking with an anesthesiologist the day before an operation:

Patient: I've heard your recommendations that I have spinal anesthesia rather than a general for my operation, but I still don't want it.

Anesth: There is something about spinal anesthesia that is frightening to you.

Patient: That long spinal needle scares me. What if it should puncture a blood vessel and cause a hemorrhage?

Anesth: You're worried that the needle might penetrate a blood vessel.

Patient: The more I think about it, I don't like the thought of being awake during the operation.

Anesth: You would rather be asleep so you won't know what is going on.

Patient: Can that be arranged?

Anesth: Yes, we can keep you asleep with very mild sedation.

Patient: Good. Let's go ahead with the spinal but with me asleep.

In this example of Active Listening, the anesthesiologist helped the patient get in touch with his deeper worry—that of being awake during surgery. He did it without advising or arguing, and he did not give further information until the patient asked for it. This is a good example of how patients can often solve their own problem better than others can advise—if only they get their feelings understood and accepted.

Physicians will have many opportunities to use Active Listening in their relationships with other members of the medical team. Following is a dialogue provided by Dr. Robert Daigneault. A problem came up when he was conducting the regular team meeting of the rehabilitation staff.

The meeting had barely started when it became obvious that the nursing staff was very upset with one patient's behavior. The patient (D.J.) was swearing at them, arguing about everything they were doing for him, and was just being very difficult to deal with. Because of his behavior, the nurses tried to have as little contact with him as possible. Thus, the patient became isolated from his primary caregivers and the nurses were becoming more angry and frustrated. The discussion went as follows:

Nurse A: I really hate going into D.J.'s room. He resents everything I do for him. Plus, he constantly swears at me. After my shift, I just want to sit down and cry.

Dr. D: You seem really upset by D.J.'s behavior.

Nurse A: Yes. I want to help him and he won't let me.

Dr. D: You want to do what you were trained to do, but his behavior gets in the way.

Nurse A: Right. I really feel sorry for him. I mean, he's paralyzed and only a teenager.

Dr. D: You feel sad because of the severity of his problems?

Nurse A: Yeah, I don't know how I would cope if I had his problems at *my* age, never mind being a teenager.

Dr. D: You are wondering how you would react in the same situation.

Nurse: Yes, I would probably be very angry and yell a lot. I probably wouldn't be nice to be around. I mean, I'd behave just like D.J.'s doing now. . . . Oh, my God. He's behaving just like I would. Wow!

Once Nurse A understood her reaction to D.J.'s behavior, she was ready to look at ways to work with D.J. without sacrificing her own feelings about him and about the situation. The two nurses who worked the other shifts caring for D.J. had experienced similar feelings, and during my exchange with Nurse A, they became more comfortable with their own feelings regarding D.J.

Another use for Active Listening is to ask patients to feedback the physician's messages so that the physician can make certain they have understood him.

K. D. Bertakis (1977) trained physicians to make a brief concluding statement at the end of their visits with patients, after which the physicians asked the patients to feedback what the physicians had said. Having the patients use Active Listening with their physicians increased their satisfaction and their recall of information given to them by their physicians.

We find this method very innovative, and we are confident that physicians could use it in a variety of situations—such as asking nurses to feedback instructions from the physicians; asking patients to feedback what they are going to do to implement agreements they made to implement the treatment regimen; asking patients to feedback educational inputs of physicians; asking patients' family members to feedback the physicians' instructions to carry out the role of caregiver for patients.

THE PROVEN BENEFITS OF ACTIVE LISTENING

The numerous benefits of the Active Listening skill are impressive. Understandably, it has sometimes been called the magical skill. In the early 1950s, its remarkable effectiveness as a tool for psychotherapists was substantiated by scores of research studies. Over the years Active Listening became an integral component in most training programs for clinical psychologists, psychiatrists, social workers, nurses, school counselors, marriage and family therapists, and personnel counselors. And it has been incorporated in most training programs for parents, teachers, and managers. It has earned its place as the best generic skill for facilitating effective two-way communication, for empowering people to solve their problems themselves, and for demonstrating empathy, understanding, and acceptance. Active Listening could in time become an essential skill for all health professionals in their relationships with patients and with each other. The benefits are numerous.

Fostering Catharsis

Many people believe their feelings will go away by suppressing them, forgetting them, or thinking about something else. Actually, people free themselves of troublesome feelings more quickly when they express them. Active Listening fosters this kind of constructive catharsis. When patients have an empathic and accepting caregiver, they feel safe to express their feelings. Equally important, they will develop positive and warm feelings toward the listener.

Facilitating Problem-Solving

We know that people do a better job of dealing with a problem when they can talk it out, as opposed to merely thinking about it. Because Active Listening is so effective in getting patients to talk, it encourages them to begin the problem-solving process for their problems. You've heard the expressions "Let me use you as a sounding board" and "Maybe it would help me if I could talk it out with you."

This is illustrated in dialogues between one of the authors (WSE) and two of his patients. The first was a stroke patient completely paralyzed in his left arm and leg and confined to a wheelchair:

WSE: What bothers you most about your problem?

Bill: I can't do home repairs, can't take RV trips, and it especially irritates me that I can't play the electric organ.

WSE: You really enjoyed playing that organ?

Bill: Yes. I was pretty good at it, too!

Nancy: He was very good. He played well and enjoyed it. [Nancy was Bill's wife.]

WSE: You had to give up something you were good at.

Bill: I tried playing with one hand, but it doesn't sound right. So I quit.

WSE: It was no fun if you couldn't do it well.

Bill: I was also a good card player, but I haven't felt like doing that since my stroke.

WSE: I wish I knew how to play card games. I never took time to learn in my earlier years.

Bill: I think I would enjoy teaching you. Why don't we try?

Sequel: Bill taught me several games, and his attitude changed dramatically during those lessons. He was enthusiastic and excited. This gave some small meaning to his life.

The second patient was a 60-year-old woman in the hospital with a neurological disease that always progresses until death in a few years. Their conversation went like this:

WSE: How are you feeling today?

Patient: I'm mad at these doctors taking care of me. They're not trying hard enough to find a cure for this disease. They're not even calling around to research centers asking what drugs they're finding that work.

WSE: You feel there must be a curative drug out there; they just aren't trying hard enough to find it.

Patient: Yes. They keep telling me there is no cure and I should just accept my fate and try to enjoy the time I have left. I'm a fighter, and I don't want to give up.

WSE: You wish they would try something new even if the chance of it working is small.

Patient: I know there's no new drug, but I don't feel these four neurologists know or care enough about me since my own neurologist retired a few months ago. I wish there was one of the four who knew my case well, so when I call their office, whoever answers doesn't have to get out my chart and read over it to find out who I am. I wish I had just one doctor who listens to my fears and my questions, and tries to learn about my rare disease.

WSE: You miss having a doctor who knows you as a person as well as a disease.

Patient: Yes, that would help a lot.

WSE: Is there some way you could make that happen?

Patient: I could ask the older doctor, the one I trust the most, if she would be my doctor. I believe I'll do that.

WSE: You would then have a knowledgeable doctor who knows you as well as your disease.

Sequel: The patient requested and received one of the neurologists as her doctor.

Reducing Fear of Feelings

"Feelings are friendly" is an expression we use in Effectiveness Training classes to help people realize that feelings are not always "bad." Again, an empathic and understanding listener who demonstrates understanding and acceptance can help patients accept feelings that they previously were afraid of or caused them shame, guilt, or anxiety.

The following dialogue illustrates the use of empathy by a physician when a mother initially refused to grant consent for her son to have a diagnostic lumbar puncture when meningitis was suspected clinically.

Physician: What concerns you about the spinal tap?

Mother: I refuse to give consent.

Physician: [*remaining calm and showing genuine interest*] Tell me more about why you are worried.

Mother: I think my son will get better without that long needle.

Physician: You are concerned about the length of the needle. [*The physician reflects to the mother her concern about the needle; this conveys to her his understanding of the problem. He purposefully avoids lecturing about the known safety of the needle.*]

Mother: Yes, I am concerned. It could make him bleed into his back.

Physician: What do you mean? [*Again, the physician tries to understand the fear rather than repeat his explanation of the procedure.*]

Mother: My neighbor's father had a bad time with headaches after a spinal tap, and Johnny is sick enough already.

Physician: So you don't want your sick child to suffer more discomfort. It is difficult for you to put him in that painful situation. [*The physician must not only understand the fear but also verbalize that understanding to the parent so that the parent knows the physician understands.*]

Mother: Yes, I'm confused. Maybe it wouldn't hurt him like it did my neighbor's father. How long is the needle? [*Now the mother relaxes and is able to listen to the physician and follow his advice.*] (Bellet and Maloney, 1991, p. 1831–32)

The following reconstruction of another clinical situation illustrates how taking a few minutes to empathize with a grandmother contributed to early diagnosis, proper treatment, and a significant reduction in cost.

A 9-year-old boy was brought to the pediatric clinic by his 72-year-old grandmother, his only caretaker. His chief complaint was recurrent abdominal pain occurring two to three times a week for the past three months. The periumbilical pain lasted an hour or two. It was not related to meals and did not prevent him from going to school or participating in his usual activities, nor did it awaken him from sleep. Otherwise, he was a healthy child with no history of major illness. The results of his physical examination were normal, as were those of the stool guaiac test. His grandmother was anxious and depressed about his problem, and barely able to cope. The following dialogue took place.

Grandmother: I am very upset about this pain and wonder if I can cope with him much longer. [*She looks anxious and angry.*]

Physician: I know you are upset and worried. You try your best and still the problem remains. [*The physician empathizes with her fear and avoids false reassurance.*]

Grandmother: Yes. I do the best I can. You know he always wants new toys and clothes from the stores. If I can't buy them, he complains that his stomach hurts. I have a limited income and can't buy everything he wants.

Physician: I understand that you're concerned about his pain. It seems to me that when he doesn't get what he wants, he develops this pain, which is real, but it occurs because he wants attention from you so that he can get what he wants.

Grandmother: Now that I think about it, I think that's it. [*She begins to relax with the physician.*] (Bellet and Maloney, 1991, p. 1832)

In this example, empathic history taking led to an in-depth understanding of the problem that relieved the grandmother's anxiety. In such cases, empathy can reduce costs by leading to early diagnosis and efficient treatment planning, thereby avoiding the spiraling costs of unnecessary and often inappropriate medical tests, prescriptions, and even hospitalizations.

Keeping Ownership of the Problem with a Patient

Active Listening communicates that the listener is not going to take over responsibility for solving the patient's problem, in contrast to giving advice, asking for information, giving logical arguments, and ordering and directing. Consequently, Active Listening is one of the most effective skills for helping people learn to think for themselves and be more self-directing and self-responsible—less dependent on others. Active Listening helps empower others, which raises their self-esteem.

Carl Rogers offered these questions to encourage helping professionals to keep responsibility with the one being helped:

Do we respect [the other person's] capacity and his right to self-direction, or do we basically believe that his life would be best guided by us? To what extent do we have a need and a desire to dominate others? Are we willing for the individual to select and choose his own values, or are our actions guided by the conviction (usually unspoken) that he would be happiest if he permitted us to select for him his values and standards and goals? (Rogers, 1951, p. 20)

Being heard by an empathic, understanding, and accepting listener feels so good that it usually generates warm and loving feelings toward the listener. There is also a reciprocal effect on the listener, because putting oneself into the shoes of another greatly increases the *listener's* understanding and valuing of that person. As a professional counselor the author (TG) often experienced becoming increasingly more caring of his clients as a result of understanding them by Active Listening—learning what each was like, why they had done the things they did, how they felt. Each subsequent counseling hour brought a deeper appreciation of each clients' uniqueness and more understanding of why he or she had developed problems. Health professionals will develop the same caring feelings toward their patients when they learn and use the skill of Active Listening. And patients will return the same kind of positive feelings toward their caregivers.

When one listens empathically and accurately to another, one gets to understand that person more, to appreciate his or her way of looking at the world—in a sense, one *becomes* that person during the period of putting oneself in the other's shoes. Invariably, by allowing oneself to "get inside" the other person, one gets feelings of closeness, caring, and love. To empathize with others is to see them as separate, yet be willing to join with them as partners. It means becoming a companion for a brief period in that person's journey through life. Such an act involves deep caring and love.

The point is movingly expressed by an Indian woman who speaks from her ancient traditions in this Shoshone poem:

> Oh, the comfort, the inexpressible comfort
> of feeling safe with a person
> Having neither to weigh thought, nor measure words,
> But pouring them all right out, just
> as they are, chaff and grain together
> Certain that a faithful hand will take and sift them;
> Keep what is worth keeping, and, with a breath
> of kindness, blow the rest away.

Carol Montgomery, R.N., describes this same caring effect when nurses put themselves in the shoes of their patients:

> When we care, we expand our consciousness so that our notion of self includes another person and consequently all other persons. . . . Connecting at this level allows us to become deeply involved with, and even love our [patients] without succumbing to destructive types of overinvolvement. (Montgomery, 1991, p. 40)

In a case study involving primary nurses and patients, it was found that patients identified the most important nursing actions as "being there" and "taking the time to sit down and listen." Findings indicated that the nurses' empathy positively influenced patients' satisfaction with their care. Another finding of interest is that nurses identified their empathic approach to patient care as what most accounted for their own satisfaction with nursing (Brown, 1990).

Another study of intensive care unit nurses found that the nurses who were more empathic showed greater ability to assess accurately the needs of ICU patients' family members (Murphy, 1992).

Dr. Ron Anderson, chief executive officer of Parkland Hospital in Dallas, talks about the environment of the hospital with Bill Moyers:

Anderson: Traditionally, hospitals have been organized for doctors, for auxiliaries, for insurance companies—everybody but the patient. . . . The total institution is like a concentration camp or jail . . . a place that was created to service a need, but that is overwhelmed with volume and stress and pain and people not dealing with their own feelings. . . . You try to bring healing to a person and help them heal themselves. Many times, if they have information, and if they're empowered through a caring milieu, they will be better able to function. The doctors and nurses won't be going home with them, so it's very important that we get them to the highest plane of function that we can. We have a saying in our geriatric ward that we've never met a patient we couldn't care for. We've met many we couldn't cure.

Moyers: Caring is good medicine.

Anderson: Yes, I think caring is a good medicine. It was good medicine when my mother gave it to me. It was good medicine back before we had antibiotics, when doctors cared, and were empathic, and talked to people. I'm afraid the technology, the wonderful drugs, and the power we have now sometimes substitute for the attitude of caring. (Moyers, 1993, p. 31)

Nurse Carol Montgomery also sees the deeper benefits of empathic listening:

So when we expand our sense of self to include another, we become part of a greater unity, liberating ourselves and our clients from the prison of isolation . . . when we allow someone to become part of our hearts, helping to heal them heals our hearts as well. (Montgomery, 1991, p. 40)

Preventing Malpractice Suits

Building mutually caring relationships between patients and health professionals will be a strong deterrent against malpractice suits, in addition to adding enjoyment to the professional life of physicians, nurses, and other caregivers. In a study to determine what brings on litigious feelings toward physicians, its authors conclude:

The results of our study support the idea that physicians may be able to affect their risk of lawsuits by changing the way they behave with patients. The use of good communication behaviors, for example, may not be technically more "competent" medicine, but it may prevent lawsuits, even when something has clearly gone wrong and even when it is clearly the physician's fault.... The positive results of the present study suggest that attempts to lower litigation risk by using extra medical procedures and tests, consultation, and extensive documentation, often known as "defensive medicine," may miss the point. Although such efforts may be preventive in that their "double-checking" may help to avoid some bad medical results, they will not prevent them all. Defensive medicine is not so much a tool to prevent lawsuits as it is to win them if they do occur. It can help provide the necessary courtroom evidence that a physician provided an appropriate standard of care. But if the intention is to prevent a lawsuit in the first place, forging a physician–patient bond that can effectively resist the pressures of our litigation-crazed and socially antagonistic society seems indispensable. An important way of accomplishing this may be through improving physician communication skills and patient education. (Lester and Smith, 1993, p. 272)

Acceptance Fosters Change

It is one of those simple but lovely paradoxes of life that when individuals feel they are truly accepted by another *as they are*, then they are freed to move from there and begin to think about *how they want to become*—how they can be different, how they might become more of what they are capable of being. Unfortunately, most of us have been brought up to believe that the best way to help people become better in the future is to tell them what it is about them in the present you don't like. We know better now. Showing unacceptance of others by trying to change them frequently closes them up, makes them uncomfortable, provokes defensiveness, deters them from looking at themselves, and thwarts constructive change.

Strong Feelings Get Defused

When listeners respond to strong feelings with Active Listening, those feelings tend to diminish in strength—the bomb that might have produced a destructive explosion and endangered a relationship is defused. People free themselves of troublemaking feelings when they are encouraged to express them openly to an accepting listener. Active Listening, then, is a powerful defusing skill. We have often seen frighteningly strong feelings disappear, simply as a result of a few moments of Active Listening. Caregivers of all professions will find this skill invaluable in dealing with strong feelings patients experience during an illness. Active Listening is particularly invaluable for dealing with the feelings of dying patients, their friends, and their relatives.

Active Listening can be very effective in dealing with troublesome patients who typically express their feelings in strongly coded messages that trigger negative responses:

What in the world are you doing that for?

Why can't I get some service on this ward?

What evidence do you have to support that idea?

What does PSA 12 mean to me?

Why don't you tell me *all* the facts?

Don't baby me; I can do it myself.

Health professionals can learn to refrain from responding to the code and focus instead on feeding back the patient's feelings or needs, as in these examples of Active Listening:

You want me to keep you informed.

You're unhappy with the service here.

You want proof that it works.

You'd like an explanation of the PSA test that you can understand.

You don't want me to hold back any information.

You'd much prefer to do these things yourself.

Active Listening to such incendiary messages of "bad" patients will communicate your acceptance of their gripes, criticisms, needs, or demands.

Patients Will Be Willing to Listen to You

Patients will be more willing to listen to and accept their physicians' or nurses' inputs if they previously have felt understood and accepted by them. This reciprocal effect of Active Listening will produce more two-way communication in the relationship with patients, and it will help make the relationship more of an equal partnership.

GUIDELINES FOR USING ACTIVE LISTENING

- Use Active Listening especially when you hear a feeling, a gripe, a disappointment, a fear; and also when you perceive that patients might want to talk about something. It's usually inappropriate and can be irritating to use Active Listening when patients are having problem-free conversations about the weather, current events, work, vacation plans, baseball scores, etc.

- Use Active Listening to help patients only when you're in a listening mood and have the time. If you're feeling rushed or impatient, or are preoccupied with your own problems, your listening won't come across as *genuinely* accepting and empathic. And it won't be accurate listening. Also make good use of the Attending Postures, Passive Listening, and Door Openers. Not every statement from the other person needs an Active Listening feedback. Use Active Listening primarily when feelings are expressed and the other person's need to be heard is unmistakable.

- Sometimes it is clearly appropriate to give patients information they need. However, first be sure you have listened long enough to be certain you understand what the patient's basic need is and what information might be most appropriate. However, don't be surprised if patients reject information or suggestions you offer.

- Avoid parroting, which is using the patient's own words (the code) to restate his or her message. Put your feedback in your own words.

- Don't *impose* Active Listening on the other person. Be sensitive to cues that the person you're trying to help doesn't want to pursue a problem and wants to stop talking about it.

- Don't use Active Listening in a manipulative way—wanting to get specific information to use later against the patient.

- Don't use Active Listening to avoid disclosing your own feelings or opinions.

- Don't fall into the habit of always starting your Active Listening with such common phrases as "Sounds like you . . . " or "I hear you saying . . . " If you do, others will begin to feel your listening is mechanical, perhaps even insincere.

- Don't expect patients to arrive at some preferred solution you have in mind. Active Listening is a tool for helping people find their own unique solutions.

- Don't expect (or insist) that patients will arrive at a solution every time. A solution may not emerge until later, and sometimes patients may never tell you how they eventually resolved a problem, thanks to your empathic listening.

CHAPTER SUMMARY

Using the consultant–client relationship as the model for collaborative relationships, we have described the critical requirements of building nonpower, nonhierarchical relationships with patients. We first focused on the initial clinical interview and then on later stages of the partnership, when patients experience various kinds of problems—such as the way they are treated, their regrets about being sick, their feelings of dependence and lack of control, their doubts about the accuracy of the diagnosis, their fear of certain treatment procedures, their worries about their family, and so on.

To build collaborative relationships with patients, it will usually be incumbent on physicians to take the initiative to describe the kind of relationship they want, to invite the patients to begin by describing their medical problems as they perceive them. Then the task of the physician is to facilitate patients' expressing themselves by being empathic, under-standing, and accepting. The one operational behavior that will most convincingly demonstrate these attitudes to patients is the skill of Active Listening. This unique communication behavior can be easily described and taught, but it takes practice to do it well.

Although using Active Listening is most critical in the initial phase of building collaborative relationships with patients, it is also appropriate and extremely effective for helping patients throughout the relationship, particularly when patients experience problems and express feelings. In fact, in helping relationships, Active Listening is an all-purpose skill that yields numerous benefits for the patient, for the health professional, and for their relationship.

Chapter 4

Roadblocks to Patient Communication

He must be a humble man to resist the temptations of a position with
so much built-in authority. The more he becomes identified with his
profession and the more he views himself as the representative of a
trained elite, the less likely he may be to see his client as someone who
is similar to him.

—Robert Katz, *Empathy—Its Nature and Uses*

The last chapter focused on a specific communication skill that has a
remarkable capability for facilitating self-disclosure of persons when they
want to talk—to express a thought, a feeling, a need, or a problem. Active
Listening involves both hearing the sender's words and actively feeding
back the listener's understanding of the meaning of those words. It is a way
of listening that has three important functions: (1) it confirms whether the
listener has understood the meaning of the sender's message; (2) it conveys
empathy for and acceptance of the sender; and (3) it encourages and often
deepens communication from the sender.

In this chapter the focus is on forms of communication and behaviors
that do not convey empathy or acceptance, and consequently discourage or
block patient communication with health professionals. What should health
professionals avoid saying or doing? What are the barriers to active patient
participation in the dialogue with physicians and other health professionals?

Some of the barriers have acquired the name Communication Road-blocks because they have been shown to block self-disclosing communication in one-to-one relationships and in groups. In "helping" or "therapeutic" relationships, where one person is trying to help another, the Roadblocks are generally not helpful or therapeutic at all—they block communication, inhibit constructive change, and impede a person's problem-solving.

Research on the communication habits of health professionals in their relationships with patients has shown extensive use of practices that both discourage and restrict patients' participation. One investigation discovered a number of behaviors that physicians employed to limit or prevent patient talk:

- Using highly technical language that turned patients off
- Clock-watching or watching the waiting list
- Mumbling to convey to the patient that the physician is thinking about the medical problem and shouldn't be interrupted
- Cutting off or interrupting the patient, sometimes by finishing the patient's sentence
- Executing a quick getaway without telling patient the visit has ended
- Ignoring a patient's question
- Showing signs of not being receptive, such as frowning.

Visits with patients were labeled as *facilitating* when the above behaviors were infrequent and as *hindering* when they were frequent. In the facilitating visits, half of the patients asked three or more questions. However, in the hindering visits, fewer than 10% asked a similar number of questions. The investigator found that physicians talked as though their patients understood them, and patients responded as though they understood the physician. In only 15% of the visits did patients tell the physician they didn't understand a term. Fear of appearing ignorant was the reason most frequently given by the patients (Svarstad, 1974).

Another barrier to patient communication stems from the dehumanizing training experience of interns and residents, which is heavily weighted toward the biochemical and technological component, as opposed to the humanistic component, of their relationships with patients. Communication skills and relating to patients take a back seat in the training of young physicians in favor of a disease-centered focus (Mizrahi, 1986).

THE TWELVE COMMUNICATION ROADBLOCKS

Early in his professional career, when he began interpersonal skill training with groups of parents, teachers, and managers, the author (TG) identified 12 potential communication blockers, which he labeled Communication Roadblocks. These were almost universally used by participants when someone expressed a feeling or began talking about a problem. Instead of listening or encouraging further communication, they invariably responded with one or more of the following messages of their own:

1. Ordering, directing, commanding
2. Warning, admonishing
3. Moralizing, preaching
4. Name-calling, labeling
5. Judging, blaming
6. Disagreeing, contradicting, teaching
7. Agreeing, supporting, praising
8. Analyzing, interpreting
9. Reassuring, sympathizing
10. Ignoring, diverting, withdrawing, interrupting
11. Questioning, probing
12. Advising, giving solutions.

Invariably persons who disclose their feelings or problems respond to these Roadblocks by not participating in any kind of problem-solving, or they stop self-disclosing altogether and direct their focus to the roadblocking message. This effect will be illustrated for each of the twelve Roadblocks, with a hypothetical patient as the sender and a health professional as the receiver and responder.

1. Ordering, Directing, Commanding

Patient: I hate doing those exercises, and besides, I don't think they're doing any good.

Physician: Keep doing them without fail, until I say you can stop. Let me be the judge.

Clearly, power-based responses like this show neither empathy for the patient nor acceptance of her strong feeling. Such responses very frequently stop further communication immediately, denying the physician any chance of learning why the patient doubts the effectiveness of the exercises, which is often the *real* problem. Such responses convey that the physician wants to be in charge, so they have no place in a consensual and collaborative relationship. Orders, directives, and commands are typically employed by authoritarians who do possess authority (power), but they are certainly inappropriate for health professionals, who don't have that kind of authority over their patients. These responses, therefore, carry a high risk of making patients feel they are being treated much like a child. Most patients resent such controlling commands and dislike the person who uses them.

2. Warning, Admonishing, Threatening

Patient: I wonder if I'll ever get over this weakness in my legs.

Nurse: If you give up hope, you'll not get well for sure.

Messages in this category certainly don't convey empathy or acceptance of the patient's pessimistic feeling. Like orders and commands, this Roadblock also can cause resentment and resistance. Patients are likely to respond to warnings and threats with an attitude of "How do you know?" or "Who says so?" This Roadblock also is commonly used by people who do have authority (power) over others—such as parents, teachers and bosses.

3. Moralizing, Preaching

Patient: I don't want to have chemotherapy. I hear it makes you very sick and it doesn't usually work.

Physician: You should go ahead with it for your husband's sake.

Telling patients what they should or ought to feel or do is seldom helpful. Such messages bring to bear on others the pressure of some external and often unknown authority—duty, obligation, religion. People frequently respond to such "shoulds," "oughts," and "musts" by resisting and defending their own postures even more strongly. These messages can communicate to patients that you do not trust their ability to judge ideas and values for themselves, so they should accept what others deem right. They may also cause feelings of guilt in patients. Moralizing messages do not communicate empathic understanding and acceptance. In fact, they convey criticism ("You ought to know better"). Like other authority-based responses, these have a high risk of blocking further communication and bruising the relationship, since they convey that the patient is not as wise as the moralizer or preacher.

4. Name-calling, Labeling

Patient: Why can't I walk to the toilet instead of using this stupid bedpan?

Nurse: Listen to Mr. Macho. Can't accept being bedridden.

These responses are bound to make patients feel foolish, inferior, or wrong. Such messages can have very damaging effects on the patient's self-image. People most frequently respond to them by being defensive: "I'm not macho." Name-calling can provoke so much defensiveness that patients respond by arguing and fighting back rather than taking a close look at themselves. These commonly employed responses have a high risk of irritating patients by putting them down rather than conveying acceptance and empathy.

5. Judging, Blaming

Patient: I feel so guilty about gaining so much weight since my last visit.

Physician: You have nobody to blame but yourself for eating so many fatty foods.

Hearing others' problems often tempts us into making negative judgments or evaluations of them. These messages, probably more than any of the others, will make patients feel defensive, inadequate, inferior, stupid, unworthy, or bad. Criticisms and negative evaluations also help shape others' self-concepts. As we judge others, so will they often judge themselves. Negative criticism also evokes countercriticism: "Then why haven't you put me on a strict diet?" Negative evaluations will strongly influence patients to keep their feelings to themselves. They quickly learn that it isn't safe to reveal their problems and share their troubles. People hate to be judged negatively, so they usually respond defensively to protect their self-images. Often they become angry and feel hostile toward the blamer, especially if the evaluation happens to be correct.

6. Disagreeing, Contradicting, Teaching

Patient: I'm too scared to have a hysterectomy. It will make me depressed. I won't be sexy anymore.

Physician: You're wrong about both of those ideas. Let me give you the facts.

These are attempts to influence the patient with facts, counterarguments, logic, information, or your own strong opinions. When you take on such a persuasive role, it's difficult to stop instructing or using arguments, yet this kind of "teaching" often makes patients feel you're seeing them as inferior, subordinate, or inadequate. Logic and facts often make others very defensive and resentful. People seldom like to be shown they're wrong. Usually it makes them defend their positions even more strongly. They often go to great lengths to discount your "facts." They may even ignore your facts and assume an "I don't care what others say" attitude. Heavy pushing doesn't build warm relationships with patients, nor does it encourage patients to keep talking.

7. Agreeing, Supporting, Praising

Patient: The older my husband gets, the more absent-minded and forgetful he gets. Drives me crazy.

Nurse: People do lose their memory when they get older. Naturally, it's going to be irritating for you.

We often think that a positive evaluation or agreement will help people feel better, keep talking, and get over their problems. Contrary to the common belief that such support is always beneficial, it often has very negative effects on a person with negative feelings and problems. A positive evaluation that does not fit the other person's self-image may also evoke denial. If you tell a cancer patient that he looks stronger when he complains about losing strength, he may see it as an insincere response.

People also infer that if we can judge them positively, we can just as easily judge them negatively some other time. Also, if praise is frequent, its absence may be interpreted as criticism.

Praise is often felt to be manipulative, a subtle way of influencing others to do what you want them to do: "You're just saying that so I'll work harder." Compliments frequently embarrass people, especially when given in front of others. And if you praise a lot, you run the risk of making people so dependent on your praise that they cannot function without constant approval from you. Agreeing with a person often stops further communication.

8. Interpreting, Analyzing

Patient: I just feel I'm steadily going downhill.

Nurse: Now, Mr. Hagler, you're just saying that to get out of taking your walk today.

Such responses tell others what you think their motives are or why they're doing or saying something. Analyzing can communicate that you think you have them all figured out and can diagnose their motives, which can be very threatening to patients. If the analysis is accurate, which it rarely is, the patient may feel embarrassed at being "exposed." If the analysis is wrong, the patient could become hurt, angry, and resistant. When we play the role of amateur psychoanalyst and analyze and interpret, we often communicate to others that we think we are superior to them. Such messages usually block further communication from others, and they are very likely to damage relationships with patients.

9. Reassuring, Sympathizing

Patient: I miss my family. I'm so lonely here.

Hospice worker: But you've made a lot of new friends here, and everyone really likes you.

Reassurance and sympathy are used far too much in dealing with patients. It is very tempting to try to make others feel better by talking them out of their feelings, minimizing their difficulties, denying the seriousness of their problems. Such messages are not as helpful as most people think. To reassure patients when they are in pain, depressed, or feeling discouraged may only convince them that you don't really understand. ("You wouldn't say that if you knew how strongly I felt.")

We often reassure others because we're uncomfortable with hearing their strong negative feelings; they give *us* pain, so we want to avoid hearing them. Such messages tell others that you can't accept what they are feeling so bad about. Also, people can easily interpret reassurances as a subtle and indirect attempt to change them.

Reassuring and consoling may imply that the troubled person could be exaggerating. If a nurse said, "Oh, you'll be just fine. You'll breeze right through this because you handle things so well," the patient could feel the nurse doesn't understand, thinks she is not in touch with reality, or is minimizing or trivializing the patient's problem. Most people throughout their lives have heard so much reassuring and sympathizing that conveyed discomfort with their feelings or nonacceptance, it's understandable they would read the same attitudes when they get reassurances from nurses, physicians, and other caregivers.

10. Ignoring, Diverting, Withdrawing, Interrupting

Patient: All my life I've taken care of myself. I get depressed being so dependent on others.

Physician: Let's take your blood pressure today, Mr. Erickson. How's that cough?

This category includes messages that convey a strong desire to withdraw or a wish to distract the person from the problem through ignoring, kidding, or changing the subject. Such messages clearly communicate lack of interest in the way the patient is, here and now. They also convey lack of respect for a person's feelings. Patients are generally quite serious and intent when they get the courage to talk about their feelings. If they hear a response that diverts or ignores them, it can make them feel hurt, rejected, belittled, frustrated—perhaps angry. Putting patients off or diverting their feelings may for the moment appear successful, but unacknowledged feelings do not always go away. Psychotherapists have proven that feelings not acknowledged and accepted often come up again and again. When physicians fail to acknowledge messages of patients and proceed to ask another question or change the subject, that can seriously bruise the relationship.

11. Questioning, Probing

Patient: I think you should be aware of how the nurses in this hospital neglect patients. I think they forget I'm here.

Physician: Do you use your call button? And have you complained to
   them?

When patients' messages clearly indicate they are having some kind of
a problem that is generating strong feelings, then probing questions can be
strong roadblocks as well as hurt the patient relationship. Probing questions
ignore the feeling the patient is experiencing, which can be interpreted by
the patient as lack of understanding or of caring. In fact, probing questions
are often consciously used when one doesn't want to deal with a person's
feelings. Probing questions also convey that the questioner is taking over
the problem—gathering the relevant facts to help find a solution rather than
using Active Listening to facilitate the patient's own problem-solving
process. When physicians ask probing questions in response to a patient's
feeling or need, it clearly structures who is in charge—who is assuming the
major responsibility for solving the patient's problem. Consequently, probing questions may seriously inhibit patient participation in the problem-
solving process.

Probing questions carry another risk. They are often irrelevant and off
target because the physician doesn't know enough about the patient's
problem to pick relevant questions. Because of this, the physician has to
resort to trial-and-error questioning. This could waste a lot of time in a
clinical interview as well as irritate the patient.

Not only do probing questions shift the locus of responsibility from
patient to physician but they severely limit the patient's area of freedom to
talk about whatever he or she feels is relevant and important. A physician's
question "When did you notice the pain?" limits the patient's answer only
to the time the pain was noticed—nothing else. "Have you been getting up
at night to urinate?" limits the patient's response to "Yes" or "No." Someone
once wisely observed, "If you ask people closed-ended probing questions,
all you get is an answer, nothing more." In other words, probing questions
program the patient's next message as clearly as if the physician said, "I
don't want to hear anything else from you other than the answer to what I
just asked." It is quite possible that many patients might want to talk about
other relevant aspects of their problem—such as how they slept last night
or how many times they go to the bathroom at night, how it produces pain,
and so on. No wonder probing questions are usually answered as briefly as
possible—often with only one word: "OK," "Yes," "No," "Fine," "Three."

Following is a disease-centered interview by a doctor in which closed-
ended probing questions are used almost exclusively, resulting in very
limited patient communication. Notice how the doctor stays in charge,

frequently roadblocks the patient, and misses opportunities to convey empathy and acceptance (Levenstein et al., 1989, p. 114).

A 68-year-old male patient, who has recently has surgery for a benign stricture of the sigmoid colon, presents for a routine follow-up office visit. The patient, a retired Roman Catholic priest, has recently moved into a retirement home for aging clergy. These facts are known to the doctor.

The Disease Centered Interview

Doctor: Hello, Father Smith, how are you today?

Patient: Fine—except for my headaches . . . (EXPECTATION)

Doctor: . . . and your operation, how's that going? (CUT-OFF)

Patient: Fine.

Doctor: Bowels working?

Patient: Yes.

Doctor: Appetite?

Patient: A bit poorly.

Doctor: Have you lost any weight? (EXPLORING THE DISEASE FRAMEWORK)

Patient: No.

Doctor: Well, obviously your loss of appetite hasn't affected anything, so it can't be too bad. . . . Any nausea or vomiting? (CUT-OFF)

Patient: None.

Doctor: Any pain at the operation site?

Patient: Not really.

Doctor: Are you eating the bran we recommended?

Patient: No.

Doctor: You must please stick to our recommendations. We don't want any recurrences.

Patient: (Sighing) Yes. (PROMPT)

Doctor: Good, well the operation seems to have been a success and there don't seem to be any complications. Have you any other complaints?

Patient: I have this headache. (PROMPT)

Doctor: Is your vision affected? (EXPLORING THE DISEASE FRAMEWORK)

Patient: No.

Doctor: Any weakness or paralysis of your limbs?

Patient: No.

Doctor: Where are your headaches?

Patient: At the back of my head.

Doctor: Do they throb?

Patient: Yes.

Doctor: How long do they last?

Patient: About four hours.

Doctor: What takes them away?

Patient: I just lie down.

Doctor: How often do they come?

Patient: About twice a week.

Doctor: How long have you been having them?

Patient: Ever since I've been at home. (PROMPT)

Doctor: Good, well, you needn't worry—it can't have anything to do with your operation. They are tension headaches. Perhaps we can give you some paracetamol for them. The home you have just moved into seems to have beautiful gardens. (CUT-OFF)

Patient: Yes.

Doctor: It really is good of the church to care for its elderly and it must be comforting to have company.

Patient: Yes.

Doctor: Well, good. Come and see me in a month's time and we'll see how things are going. Take care.

Closed-ended questions also may come across to patients as manipulative. Our experiences with salespeople have conditioned us to feel trapped by their leading questions, such as this one from a salesperson selling before-need cemetery plots: "Would you want your wife to have to deal with all these emotional problems and make all these decisions in the few days after you have passed away?"

Health professionals need to avoid such leading questions, because they can put patients out on a limb and induce guilt and defensiveness. For example: "Do you ever count your calories, Mr. Taylor?"

People often feel threatened by probing questions, especially when they don't understand *why* they are being questioned. Recall how people so often answer a probing question with a question of their own such as these: "Why are you asking?" "Do you suspect I might have diabetes?" "Are you thinking that I shouldn't take aspirin so often?"

Are there alternatives to closed-ended probing questions? Certainly Active Listening is one—and a very effective one. It will convey acceptance and empathic understanding, it keeps the locus of responsibility with the patient, it stimulates more self-disclosure, and it often paves the way for patients to get down to a more basic or underlying problem.

A second alternative to probing questions is open-ended questions, which have a high probability of eliciting much more information from patients:

What are you experiencing during the night?

How would you describe the pain you experience?

Why do you think you have headaches only at home?

What has been your experience since our last visit?

How are things going after your operation?

What do you think your loss of appetite could be caused by?

Can you think of anything else that may be relevant?

Such questions will elicit much more information, and they will give health professionals more opportunities for using Active Listening to convey empathy, understanding, and acceptance.

One study showed that physicians who used a "high control interviewing style" asked a lot of probing closed-ended questions, and they rarely used open-ended questions. The visits of 50 new patients with 20 family practice residents were audiotaped. After eliciting family information, the residents missed numerous opportunities to express empathy or verbal concern. The physicians seldom connected information about the patient's family with the patient's ongoing or potential health problem. It was concluded that probing and the closed-ended style of interviewing appeared to interfere with the physicians' gathering and responding to important family information (Crouch and McCauley, 1986).

The research of Roter and Hall (1987) found that open-ended questions provided physicians substantially more relevant information from patients than closed-ended questions. They support the use of open-ended questions to foster more information exchange in a two-way process:

> Patients spend most of their time during the medical visit providing information to physicians—largely in response to physicians' questions (mostly closed-ended) about the medical condition. But this kind of information is incomplete. Giving patients the opportunity to tell their story in an open manner, with minimal direction by the physician, can increase both provider and patient understanding of the patient's condition and his or her experience. The reflection and insight that can arise from the telling of the story can move the level of exchange to a deeper and more meaningful interaction. (Roter and Hall, 1992, p. 105)

In yet another study of physicians' methods for soliciting patients' information and concerns about their health problem, investigators found that among the linguistic responses that produced interruption of patients' statements, closed-ended questions were most frequent (46%). A most striking finding was that only one of 52 interrupted opening patient statements was subsequently completed, even though there was no audible evidence that the patient had finished answering the question "What problems are you having?" (Beckman and Frankel, 1984).

There may be times, however, when closed-ended probing questions may be appropriate and effective. Such questions are sometimes defended as a way of testing a diagnostic hypothesis, the questions serving as prompts to the patient to give the physician the information needed. This method of doing differential diagnosis is obviously a disease-centered approach and at times may be appropriate. If such closed-ended questions are needed, physicians should be encouraged to explain this to their patients, telling them the purpose of the closed-ended questions:

1. *Physician*: I'll need now to ask some quick questions to help us find out what kind of headaches you're having.

2. *Physician*: There are several different indications of an enlarged prostate. So now I'll need to ask you some very specific and personal questions to see how many of these symptoms you have.

Such explanations communicate to patients that the physician wants to keep them as active participants and respects them by giving reasons for temporarily taking charge. These explanations help reconcile the patient-centered clinical interview and the disease-centered framework.

Dr. Thomas Delbanco, when interviewed by Bill Moyers, had this to say about using the typical disease-centered interviewing approach, which he called the "doctor's review" system, in conjunction with a patient-centered approach:

Delbanco: That's what I can do in my sleep, standing on my head, having been up all night, and having drunk too much wine. I can do the review of systems, going from your heart to your gastro-intestinal tract to your kidneys to your this and that—it's a patter song. I learned it first thing in medical school, and I'll always be able to do it. What we don't ask and what I'd like to see us ask is how is Bill Moyers different from other people?

Moyers: But why do you want to know that? What difference does it make to my healing while I'm in that hospital?

Delbanco: It makes an enormous difference. It helps me talk to you in ways that are helpful to you. For example, you may want to be told everything about what's wrong with you. Or you may not want to know anything about what's wrong with you. You may want me just to say, do this, do that. You may want your family very involved in your care. Or you may want to keep your family at a distance. You may want to endure pain because you're tough, and you think it's good for you to hurt a little bit. Or you may want to feel no pain because you're afraid of pain, and it makes you sick, which might affect your response to medicines and other things. I've got to know what makes you tick. I may know a lot about your disease, but I don't know how you experience your illness. The attitude with which you confront your illness will make a real difference in how you do over time. (Delbanco, 1993, p. 13)

12. Advising, Giving Solutions

This form of communication can be a roadblock when it is a response to a message that indicates the patient has a strong feeling, a need, or a problem. It can block communication if it is advice or a solution that is unacceptable to the patient. It can also be a roadblock if the patient has already tried the solution offered by the physician or if the solution requires the patient to change what he or she has been doing and adopt a different way of behaving. Although physicians do possess Authority (Expertise), they need to know when it is appropriate to offer it and how to communicate it so that the patient's resistance will be minimal.

Studies have shown that people are more apt to accept expert advice from people whom they like and with whom they have a satisfying relationship. Patients are more likely to comply with their physician's treatment advice if they are satisfied with the relationship they have with their physician (Korsch and Negrete, 1972).

In all consultant–client relationships the use of power-based control—ordering, directing, persuading, admonishing, and so on—not only won't change client behaviors but will reduce the overall potential for influencing clients even with *nonpower* forms of communication. This is because consultant–client relationships are consensual, with the consultant having very little authority (power). In such relationships the client (or changee) is in the driver's seat. The locus of responsibility for change resides with the client. This is obviously the case with relationships between health professionals and patients. Should health professionals try to control their patients or hassle them, they will encounter overt resistance or covert noncompliance. Use power to try to control another, and you will lose influence—an interesting paradox in human relationships.

Like successful consultants, health professionals should make sure they are hired by their patients—that is, they should first ascertain that the patient is ready to accept their Authority (Expertise). Often a simple question will assess the patient's readiness for advice. For example:

Are you ready to know what I would advise?

Do we have sufficient agreement about your problem to begin considering various solutions?

I have possible solutions in mind. Are you ready to hear them?

These questions obviously give patients evidence of the willingness of their health professional to have them participate more and take more responsibility for their health.

INTERRUPTIONS

Nothing can block patients' self-disclosing communication more consistently than interrupting them before they have finished their message. Yet interrupting patient talk seems to be very common, probably because it is a manifestation of the need of many health professionals to remain in charge which may stem from their need to keep their visits with patients as short as possible.

The effects of being interrupted, as all of us have experienced, are invariably detrimental to relationships. We feel frustrated, rejected, and often angry. It can bring back early reactions we had as youngsters when adults so frequently interrupted us. It sends a message of disrespect—our thoughts and feelings are not seen as important.

Any of the Roadblocks can be used to interrupt patients. Studies show that physicians very frequently use their own questions to interrupt patients. However, one can interrupt a speaker by reassuring, contradicting, analyzing, moralizing, or advising.

The obvious remedy for interrupting is to wait until patients show evidence of having finished their messages, then use Active Listening to convey acceptance and empathic understanding. Of course, there will be times when interruptions will be justified—telephone calls, a nurse entering the examining room, and so on. No harm will be done, however, especially if the patient hears "I'm sorry for the interruption; please go ahead with what you were telling me."

There will be times in relationships with patients when the Communication Roadblocks won't block communication or harm the relationship. This is when neither patient nor health professional is expressing a feeling or sharing a problem—when both are task oriented, both are getting their needs met, both are involved in mutual problem-solving to find the best way to deal with the patient's health problem.

In Chapter 7, we will have more to say about these "on task" or "no problem" periods.

CHAPTER SUMMARY

In relationships in which one of the parties owns a problem and the other is seen as a potential helper, certain kinds of verbal messages block the helpee's self-disclosure and active participation in the relationship. Twelve such messages were identified, and their potential risks were described. These Communication Roadblocks are commonly used by health professionals, particularly closed-ended probing questions and giving advice and solutions. Suggestions were made that can help reduce the risks and negative effects of these roadblocks.

It seems appropriate to conclude this chapter on Roadblocks with a poem written by someone whose identity is unknown but whose message is clear. Although the message may not have been written by a medical patient, it is certainly applicable to all helping professionals:

Listen

When I ask you to listen to me
    and you start giving me advice,
    you have not done what I asked.
When I ask you to listen to me
    and you begin to tell me why
    I shouldn't feel that way
    you are trampling on my feelings.
When I ask you to listen to me
    and you feel you have to do something
    to solve my problem,
    you have failed me,
    strange as that may seem.
Listen! All I asked was that you listen,
    not talk or do—just hear me.
Advice is cheap; twenty cents will get
    you both Dear Abby and Billy Graham
    in the same newspaper.
And I can do for myself. I am not
    helpless.
    Maybe discouraged and faltering,
    but not helpless.
When you do something for me that I can
    and need to do for myself,
    you contribute to my fear and
    inadequacy.
But when you accept as a simple fact
    that I do feel what I feel,
    no matter how irrational,
    then I can quit trying to convince
    you and can get about this business
    of understanding what's behind
    this irrational feeling.

And when that's clear, the answers are
        obvious and I don't need advice.
        Irrational feelings make sense when
        we understand what's behind them.
Perhaps that's why prayer works,
        sometimes, for some people—because
        God is mute, and He/She doesn't give
        advice or try to fix things.
"They" just listen and let you work it
        out for yourself.
So please listen and just hear me.
And if you want to talk, wait a minute for
        your turn—and I'll listen to you.

Chapter 5

Self-Disclosure Skills for Health Care Professionals

> Assertive behavior means knowing what you need and want, making this clear to others, working in a self-directive way to get your needs met while showing respect for others.
>
> —Linda Adams, *Be Your Best*

Although relationships between health professionals and patients, like most consultant–client relationships, are created to help patients get their needs met and solve their problems, this fact doesn't mean that health professionals must ignore their own needs. Nor does it imply that health professionals won't ever experience problems in their relationships with patients. Although the role of health professionals is that of a helping agent, they are first of all human beings with human feelings. Like everyone else, they can feel tired, irritated, frustrated, sad, inadequate, hurt. Particular patients may be difficult to deal with. Also, problems outside relationships with patients may affect their mood or reduce health professionals' effectiveness. And, most important, health professionals have a strong need to do a good job—to be competent and successful.

For these reasons health professionals need special skills for getting their own needs met as well as skills for helping patients meet their needs. They need to acquire assertive skills as well as listening skills; they need effective self-disclosure skills as well as the skills to help patients self-disclose.

In this chapter, we will focus on self-disclosure skills for health professionals. Why are they needed? What benefits do they yield? What are the potential risks of disclosing one's feelings and needs? How can these risks be greatly reduced?

WHY SELF-DISCLOSE TO PATIENTS?

If health professionals commit to adopting the consensual consultant–client model for their relationship with patients, two-way communication is essential, because collaborative relationships utilize the knowledge and wisdom of *both* participants—their Authority (Expertise). And collaborative relationships value and strive for mutual need satisfaction, which requires open, honest, and direct two-way self-disclosure. Authoritarian relationships, on the other hand, don't foster two-way communication—most of it comes from the person in charge.

A less obvious reason for self-disclosing to patients is that it will promote reciprocity—self-disclosure from the patient to the health professional. Gordon Chelune, a University of Georgia psychologist, after reviewing hundreds of research studies for his book *Self-Disclosure*, concluded:

> Perhaps the most reliable and robust situational determinant of disclosure is the disclosure of another person. This "reciprocity" or "dyadic" effect has been frequently demonstrated and seems to override the influence of any individual difference variables. (Chelune, 1979, p. 246)

Psychologist Sidney Jourard, in his pioneering book *The Transparent Self*, also stressed that nurses and/or doctors who freely self-disclose to their patients will encourage their patients to self-disclose (Jourard, 1971). However, Jourard reported that his work with nurses led him to observe that their "character armor" serves to protect them from having *real* feelings—pity, anger, inadequacy, or sadness—as they relate to suffering or demanding patients. Jourard believed there was a connection between a nurse's fear of being her real self while on duty and the blocking of patients' disclosing important information needed by the nurse:

> Yet, the bedside manner [professional role] is nicely designed to exclude a highly important source of information that has much pertinence to the optimum response of the patient to treatment . . . information which can only be obtained through the patient's verbal disclosure of what is on his mind. (Jourard, 1971, p. 183)

One of the other effects of the conventional professional role is to reduce patients' disclosure of what is *really* on their minds—thoughts or feelings that could have an important bearing on their medical problem and/or their response to treatment. For example, the stereotyped optimistic role that some nurses put on when they don their uniform can reduce patient self-disclosure. Many nurses always smile, act cheerful, routinely reassure patients, using such stock phrases as "Doctor knows best," "You're going to get well," "You're looking a lot better," "Don't you worry."

Jourard also believed that nurses potentially have not just an important role in healing but possibly the *most* important role:

> If they can permit patients to be themselves in their presences and not be driven away by whatever the patients bring forth when they are thus granted freedom of self-expression; if they can communicate profoundly with patients, so that the latter overcome a profound sense of loneliness that seems to be part of illness . . . if they can help patients feel that there is someone who cares, to whom their feelings and wishes matter, they may so restore identity and morale to patients that they get well in spite of the usually impersonal regimen of hospital life. (Jourard, 1964, p. 150)

Other health professionals may also assume a stereotyped role or a professional posture that will inhibit patient self-disclosure. Obviously, health professionals can't escape the tasks and duties prescribed by their job definition, yet they are still *real persons* carrying out their prescribed tasks with other real persons. The nature of their professional training tends to encourage them to assume a professional role that limits their open and honest self-disclosure and keeps them at a safe psychological distance from patients in order to save time.

Another reason for health professionals to self-disclose is that it enables them to keep in close touch with themselves. Sociologist Linda Adams points out that openly communicating one's needs, feelings, or ideas to others is very different from merely thinking about them.

> *The act of saying something aloud transforms it.* You've probably had the experience of mulling a particular problem over and over in your mind so much that it got bigger and bigger and seemed much worse. You imagined outcomes and conjured up others' reactions. Later, when you did relate your problem to someone else, it came out in an entirely different way. (Adams, 1989, p. 38)

Self-disclosure also gives people a chance to get important needs met in their relationship, when help or cooperation from the other person is necessary. Finally, self-disclosure makes one appear to others like a real person, and a more interesting one at that. Failure to self-disclose hides one's individuality. Particularly for physicians and nurses, being seen by patients as real persons will tend to reduce the professionals' "psychological size," thus giving patients more confidence to speak up and reveal their needs and problems rather than subordinate their thoughts to those of the health professionals. Many patients have admitted going away from a visit with a physician feeling angry, frustrated, and resentful because they didn't disclose how they really felt.

In an article identifying the "communication barriers" that develop in physician–patient encounters, Dr. Timothy Quill points out the value of physicians' self-disclosing when the barrier is often caused by some problem being experienced by the physician, such as feeling bored with or detached from a patient—feelings that are often a product of overwork and lack of sleep. Quill recommends as follows:

> Depending on the patient and the nature of the relationship, the physician might openly acknowledge that she is exhausted, and suggest to the patient that the visit be more limited in time and scope than usual. Such an admission might make the physician seem more like a human being to the patient, and might allow the patient to reciprocate some of the nurturing feelings he had received from the physician in the past, thereby enhancing their relationship of mutual caring and respect. (Quill, 1989, p. 54)

Quill takes the strong position that *anything* acting as a barrier to solving the health problem of the patient should be disclosed and dealt with openly, honestly, and directly.

EFFECTIVE SELF-DISCLOSURE

Although self-disclosure *can* be beneficial in all human relationships, there is some risk that it may make the other person feel uncomfortable, hurt, or defensive. It can bruise a relationship or even end it. These risks, however, can be greatly reduced by the way people disclose their thoughts and feelings.

It may at first seem obvious, but the most effective and least risky self-disclosing messages one can send are those that only convey one's own thoughts, feelings, or needs. It follows that such effective messages will begin with the pronoun "I" or at least have a heavy component of "I", as in the following examples:

I believe we should not punish children.

I need your help today.

I get irritated when . . .

I feel very disappointed with . . .

Today, *I* feel especially tired.

I should remember that, but I don't.

I really feel bad when a patient has to wait so long.

This author (TG) coined the term "I-Message" when it became clear in his P.E.T. classes that the self-disclosures of most parents weren't really messages about themselves but instead were messages about their children. Their self-disclosures typically began with "You," as in these examples:

You stop making so much noise.

You ought to know better.

You are not thinking clearly.

You don't have the facts.

You make me worry when you're late.

Don't *you* ever hit your baby brother.

You don't know what you're talking about.

You should do what your teacher tells you to do.

The negative effects of You-Messages will be described more fully later in this chapter. For now, we will examine the four different kinds of I-Messages: Declarative, Responsive, Preventive, and Confrontive.

Declarative I-Messages

These messages share with others one's beliefs, ideas, preferences, opinions. Here are examples of the kind of Declarative I-Messages health professionals might send:

I'm excited today. My daughter graduates from college.

I'm exhausted from being on call last night.

I believe walking is safer than running.

Frankly, I'm at a loss how to explain your rather high systolic blood pressure.

I really hate to see you in so much pain.

I like coming into your room and seeing you smiling again.

I'm interested in knowing more about your family.

Responsive I-Messages

These are messages that clearly communicate how you feel when you get a request from someone. If you genuinely feel a willingness to consent to the request, there is seldom a problem. Your response will simply communicate your acceptance:

Sure, I would like to raise your bed and open the curtains; I want you to have a bright and cheery room.

I'd be happy to bring you some ice water; I'm sure it will be refreshing.

However, most people find it difficult to refuse another's request, for fear of hurting the person, provoking disapproval, or damaging the relationship. However, if one learns to respond with I-Messages, it gets much easier to refuse a request. Here are some Responsive I-Messages that clearly communicate a nurse's unwillingness to consent to patients' requests, plus a clear statement of why:

No, I don't want to bring you a painkiller, because of your physician's orders not to do that.

No, I have to refuse your request to read to you; I want to complete my duties with all my other patients.

I don't feel good about giving you more sleeping pills; I'm worried about your becoming too dependent on them.

Preventive I-Messages

Preventive I-Messages communicate your need for another person to do something that might prevent a problem for you in the future. When one has a need that will require some form of cooperation, support, or action by another, the full disclosure by the person of his or her need is a *Preventive I-Message*. It is a self-disclosure that involves a person in a shared experience with another person who can help you get your needs met. It is so named because it is a message that can effectively *prevent* many problems or conflicts by informing others ahead of time what you will need in the future. This keeps them closely involved with you, keeps them from being surprised later on, and gives them a chance to avoid behavior that otherwise would be unacceptable to you and cause you a problem. These messages are *self*-oriented as opposed to *other*-oriented. They communicate "This is what *I* will need," as opposed to "This is what *you* must or should do." Here are some examples of Preventive I-Messages in various caregiver–patient relationships.

1. *Nurse*:   I will be going to work on another ward in 15 minutes, so I would like to know now if you think you'll need me for something before I leave.

2. *Physician*:   I would like to be certain that you'll not be late for our next appointment, because our X ray machine will be tied up from 2:30 until our office closes, and I want to make sure we get a picture of that arm at your next visit.

3. *Physical Therapist*: I want you to know that you can expect some pain tomorrow from this treatment, so that you won't be frightened and wonder what's wrong.

4. *Physician*:   I would like you to write down every question that comes to you between now and our next appointment, so you'll remember to ask me what you want to know.

Notice that each of these Preventive I-Messages contains no blame, put-downs, corrections, or scolding. Instead, they communicate a desire on the part of the professional to prevent some problem *in the future*—for the benefit of either or both persons in the relationship.

Pediatrician Dr. Peggy Manuel explained to the author (TG) how she uses Preventive I-Messages with children:

When I have to give shots to pre-school kids I find a lot of them are worried about that, which I can often see when they walk into my office. I show them I don't have any needles in my hand, and I explain that if they do need a shot it will be after I leave the room, because our nurse is the one who will give the shots. If I still see that a child is worried about the shots, I'll ask them if they want to talk about it now or wait until I leave and talk to the nurse. I don't believe in giving any kind of painful procedure to the child without advance warning and an explanation where it will be given. If they want to talk about it, I usually send a Preventive I-Message such as: "I want to tell you now that if you have to get a shot, I'm certain you'll have an 'ouch' on your finger or on your arm. I would really worry about you if you weren't worried about shots, because nobody likes shots."

I feel there are a lot of opportunities for prevention with small children. I start recommending books; I examine small children in the mother's arms. Being able now to examine children without them crying is something I didn't learn until after I took the P.E.T. training. Sending children Preventive I-Messages is very helpful in preventing all kinds of problems. (Manuel, 1993)

Confrontive I-Messages

Confrontive I-Messages are those you send when a patients' behavior is interfering, or has already interfered, with your getting some need of your own satisfied. Your goal is to send a message that will influence (not compel) the patient to change the behavior that is unacceptable to you. Consequently, we need to examine these messages much more in depth than the other three types of I-Messages. Confronting patients is called for when the health professional is experiencing a negative feeling, a need, a problem, a barrier to effective communication in the relationship.

There are some special problems with confronting messages. They are the most risky in all relationships. Nevertheless, health professionals cannot avoid experiencing unacceptance of certain behaviors of their patients, and wanting to change them. Patients can be surly, demanding, forgetful, uncooperative, hypercritical. They can neglect to pay a bill, they can be rude, they can gripe about the hospital food, they can phone their physicians or call nurses too often, they can be late for appointments, they can resist conforming to hospital rules and routines, they can fail to follow their treatment regimen. It is inevitable that health professionals will find such behaviors unacceptable—behaviors that deprive or threaten to deprive them of meeting *their* needs, behaviors that give *them* a problem. They can feel angry at a demanding or otherwise difficult patient, irritated with excessive phone calls from a patient, discouraged when a patient doesn't comply with the treatment regimen, upset because a patient hasn't paid a bill, worried about a patient receiving excessive phone calls and visitors in the hospital. We found in the medical literature a variety of names for difficult patients, confirming our belief that health professionals do encounter patients whose behavior is unacceptable:

Obnoxious patients

Bad patients

Crocks

Whiners and self-pitiers

Clingers

Demanders

Help rejectors

Denying patients

Self-murderous patients

Hateful patients.

Undoubtedly, other types might be identified. However, in the particular blueprint or model for human relationships we propose, this patient-centered typology has no place at all. Rather, we strongly emphasize the importance of always thinking in terms of specific *behaviors* rather than *types of people*. Apart from our antipathy toward most typologies (which are so often invalid), it is so much easier to deal with *behaviors* you can see or hear than with generalizations of different *patients*.

THE BEHAVIOR WINDOW AND PROBLEM OWNERSHIP

We offer a graphic model that will help the reader (1) think about unacceptable *behaviors* rather than unacceptable persons, (2) understand the concept of *problem ownership* in person-to-person relationships, and (3) understand that changing another person's unacceptable behavior requires using communication skills much different from those called for when the other person has the problem and you want to help him or her.

This graphic model begins with a rectangle. Think of it as a window through which you (a health professional or caregiver) will see each and every behavior of a particular patient—what the patient does or says in your

presence. Over time you will see countless specific behaviors of the patient
through the window, each behavior represented by a B:

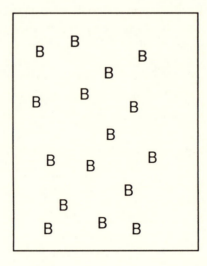

We now divide the Behavior Window into two areas. Through the top
area of the window you will see only the patient's behaviors that are
acceptable to you; in the bottom area you'll see only behaviors that are
unacceptable to you.

Acceptable
Behaviors

Unacceptable
Behaviors

Acceptable patient behaviors are those that you can genuinely accept because they do not tangibly deprive you (or threaten to deprive you) of meeting some need of yours. Unacceptable patient behaviors are those that deprive you (or threaten to deprive you) of meeting some need of yours.

Acceptable behaviors are those you like. Unacceptable behaviors you don't like—you wish they hadn't occurred and you hope they'll go away. They interfere with your doing the professional tasks you need to do as effectively as you would like.

What clues tell you that a patient's behavior is unacceptable to you? Your own feelings are obviously the most reliable clues. You find yourself dreading interacting with a patient; you get feelings of irritation or even anger with a patient; you feel bored and inattentive; you find you are seldom pleasant to a patient; you feel pushed by a patient's excessive demands on you. When you experience such feelings, the behavior of the patient, whatever it might be, is causing you a problem. Locate those behaviors in the bottom part of your Behavior Window.

You get very different clues, however, when a patient's behavior is acceptable. Now your feeling about the patient is positive, you welcome seeing the patient, you don't experience any negative effects, and you are able to direct all your attention to whatever task your job requires you to perform. And the relationship with the patient feels good.

We also need to designate a third area in the top of your Behavior Window. There you'll see behaviors that give you clues that the patient is experiencing some kind of problem or need deprivation.

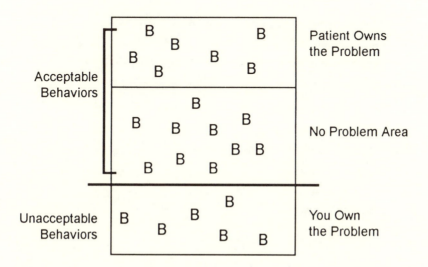

Some behavior clues will be nonverbal—for example, a patient seems quieter than usual, a patient appears to have something else on his/her mind, a patient seems tense, anxious, depressed. Or a patient may come right out and verbally inform you something is wrong: "I'm worried," "I'm discouraged," "Am I ever going to get well?" "I can't get to sleep at night," "Why did this have to happen to me?" "Why didn't you call me back?" "I have been in the waiting room 50 minutes." "Are you sure you have told me everything I should know about what's wrong with me?"

While such behaviors—verbal or nonverbal—are clues that your *patient* has a problem, those behaviors usually are not directly causing *you* a problem. In fact, you should welcome such behaviors as clues that tell you the patient has some kind of a problem, much as pain warns of the existence of some physical problem in one's body. The Behavior Window is also a visual model for highlighting an important concept—*problem ownership*. Obviously, whenever a patient's behavior is interfering (or has already interfered) with your meeting your needs or causing you to feel troubled, upset, worried, frustrated, or angry, then *you own the problem*. And whenever the patient gives off a clue or sends you a verbal or nonverbal message indicating some need deprivation, unhappiness, or dissatisfaction with what is going on, the *patient owns the problem*.

This concept of problem ownership is very important in interpersonal relationships, because a different posture and different interpersonal skills are called for, depending upon who owns the problem.

Patient Owns Problem	You Own Problem
You want to be the helper	You want to be helped
You become a listener	You become a sender
You want the patient to talk	You want to talk
You want to understand	You want to be understood
You want to be accepting	You want to be accepted
You respect the patient's needs	You respect your own needs
You take a facilitative role	You take a proactive role
You want to empower the patient to problem-solve	You want to problem-solve

The effective skills for dealing with problems owned by your patients have already been identified and illustrated in chapters 3, 4, and 5—open-ended questions, attending, Passive Listening, and Active Listening.

Now think of the middle area of your Behavior Window as representing those times when no behavior of your patient is giving you a problem, nor do you get any indication that the *patient* has a problem. This is the No Problem Area. Here are some examples of behaviors that belong in the middle area:

Nurse is hooking up an IV for a patient and the patient gives no clues that she has a problem with this.

Physician is taking a history, the patient is self-disclosing freely, and physician is getting the information needed.

Physical therapist is helping patient stretch a tight muscle and patient is not complaining that it is too painful.

Physician is prescribing a bland diet for a patient with an ulcer and patient gives no indication of reluctance to comply.

Hospice worker comes in to get patient out of bed for a walk down the hall and patient gives no evidence of resisting.

In the above situations, it is quite obvious that those health professionals are able to perform the prescribed functions and duties appropriate to the situation, and the patients are showing no dissatisfaction with what is happening. Their relationships can be described as being "on task." Obviously practitioners would prefer that all their time spent with patients would be problem-free and on task, but that doesn't always happen. So the first challenge in dealing effectively with patients and building good relationships with them is to become a sensitive observer and listener, so one can pick up clues from patients when they have problems in the relationship. The second challenge for health professionals is to become sensitively aware of their own feelings that tell them they are "owning" a problem in their relationship with the patient. The third challenge, of course, is to become competent in using the particular skills most appropriate for each of the two problem areas.

As a health professional you want to see to it that the patient's problems get acknowledged and resolved whenever they occur, and also that your problems get expressed and resolved, so that both you and the patient can get back on task. The ultimate goal is to reduce the number of problems in your relationship with each patient—both the problems *you* own and the problems the *patient* owns.

Of greatest importance is to recognize that an entirely different set of skills will be required in each of the two problem areas of the Behavior

Window, as shown below:

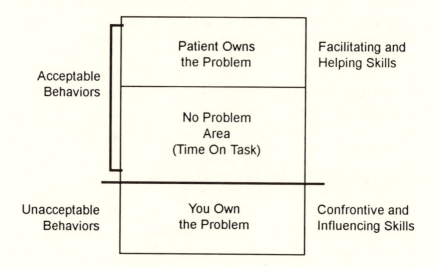

A reduction of both kinds of problems brought about by utilizing the appropriate skills can be represented in the Behavior Window by a reduction of the top and bottom areas and an enlargement of the No Problem Area. By solving the problems in the relationship, there will be much more time on task—time to practice your particular profession, whether you are a physician, nurse, or other health professional.

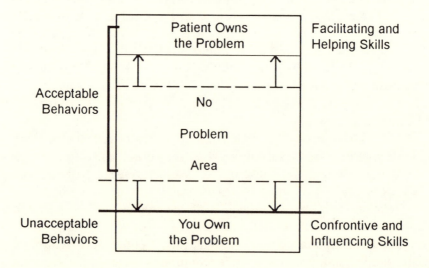

In the previous diagram, the No Problem area is shown greatly enlarged, although typically patients will still experience some occasional problems you may never be aware of or never get solved. Likewise, you might have a few problems you do not choose to communicate to the patient. Nevertheless, by using both sets of interpersonal communication skills to reduce time-consuming problems in their relationships with patients, health professionals can significantly increase the amount of time available for practicing their profession, for using their biomedical Authority (Expertise) to help patients with health problems. A benefit of additional value will be increased patient satisfaction with the health professional, who in turn will experience the personal enrichment derived from relating to each patient as a *unique person* rather than as a patient or a particular disease.

In the words of nurse Carol Montgomery, in her article "Caring vs. Curing":

It's not what we do, it's what we allow ourselves to become part of. . . . When we care, we expand our consciousness so that our notion of self includes another person and consequently all other people. . . . Nor should we fear that we will lose ourselves in the process. . . . You do not lose your identity like a drop in the ocean. . . . You become more yourself . . . when we allow someone to become part of our hearts, helping to heal them heals our hearts as well. (Montgomery, 1991, p. 40)

HIGH-RISK WAYS OF CONFRONTING PATIENTS

Most of us are very reluctant to confront other people when their behavior is unacceptable or is creating a problem for us. We are afraid the other person may feel hurt, get angry, not like us. And these fears are not unwarranted. People often do respond to confrontation with negative reactions we don't like to hear. They may walk away hurt or angry. They may start an argument. They may get defensive and disagreeable. Consequently, it takes a certain amount of courage to assert ourselves and confront others. If this courage is not forthcoming, the problem will remain, and the frustration or anger that builds up may threaten the relationship.

You-Messages

One reason why people approach the task of confronting each other with so much anxiety is that the particular language they employ, originally learned from adults who confronted *them* as children, has shown a very high probability of provoking resistance and retaliation, and sometimes bruises the relationship. As pointed out earlier, these confronting messages are typically You-Messages—messages that contain a heavy component of *you*—and they typically come across as abrasive, judgmental, blameful, threatening, moralizing, or condescending. Instead of influencing the patient to change the behavior that is unacceptable, these You-Messages, which focus on the patient, usually provoke resistance to change.

To illustrate, take the case of a nurse working in a hospital. One of the patients on the ward has been getting out of bed several times a day to go to the bathroom to smoke a cigarette. Smoking is not allowed on the ward, and the patient has not recovered enough from surgery to get out of bed without help. Following are some You-Messages the nurse might send:

Don't (*you*) leave your bed yet, and you're not to smoke.

If *you* persist in breaking the rules, I'll have to report you to your doctor.

You should consider other people's needs, not just your own.

(*You*) wait until you get home to smoke.

Let me tell *you* the effects of your walking too soon after an operation.

You are being foolish and thoughtless.

You've been a good patient up until now.

What a troublemaker *you* are.

I'll bet *you* were a rebel as a child.

It won't be hard for *you* to wait until you get home to smoke.

Why did *you* do it? Did you think you'd get away with it?

Note that the messages sent by our hypothetical nurse all contain the pronoun "you." They push the problem ownership from the nurse to the patient. The focus is on *the patient*—the You-Messages order, warn, moralize, teach, give solutions, criticize, praise, name-call, psychoanalyze, reassure, question, or humor *the patient*. In such You-Messages there is no trace of the nurse—not a single *feeling* of the nurse, no *consequences* of the patient's behavior for the nurse.

What else is wrong with You-Messages? Our experience in working with parents, teachers, and managers clearly reveals that You-Messages are high-risk messages that carry a high probability of the following:

- Provoking resistance to change

- Putting down the other person

- Making the other feel the sender has no consideration for the other's needs

- Making the other person feel blamed, guilty

- Reducing the other person's self-esteem

- Provoking strong defensiveness

- Provoking retaliation.

The first four examples of the nurse's You-Messages were solutions—what the patient *must* or *should* or *better* do. Such messages convey a lack of trust for the patient to come up with a solution.

The next four You-Messages communicate put-downs—that is, blame, judgment, ridicule, criticism. They impugn the character of the patient and underline his or her inadequacies. Even praise can come across as manipulative ("You have so much potential.").

Analyzing is seldom welcome to anyone—it conveys superiority—and implies that the nurse can see into the patient's motives. Reassuring messages seldom reassure, but they often make the other person feel "You don't really know how hard it really is." Finally, interrogating and diverting messages seldom influence others to change.

Angry Messages

A very common response to another's unacceptable behavior is *anger*. Should one express anger? The conventional wisdom, even among professionals, has been that people *should* express their anger, because it is thought to be healthy to do so. Authors write about anger as "storming and raging through one's body" or sitting in some unspecified internal organ, ever ready to pop out:

She's got a lot of anger *buried* in her.

He needs to *release* his anger.

If anger gets *blocked*, it turns inward and gets *bottled up*.

When angry, let it all *come out* so it can spend itself and be done with.

Recent studies of anger have repeatedly taken the position that one's anger is almost always a message that points the finger at the other person—a You-Message:

I'm angry at *you*.

Look what *you've* done now.

You make me so mad.

You never keep your promises, damn it!

Furthermore, anger is usually a secondary feeling, preceded by some earlier primary feeling—such as fear, embarrassment, hurt, or disappointment. In fact, anger is most often a deliberate posture, an act or a role that one assumes for the purpose of teaching the other person a lesson, getting back at him, punishing him, coercing him not to do the same thing again. We might say that when someone's behavior causes us need deprivation and evokes some primary feeling such as hurt, disappointment, or neglect, we often put on an act of being angry and send a teaching, blaming, or punishing message as noted above. *We manufacture or generate our own anger for a particular purpose*: to teach a lesson, punish, or get back at the other.

To avoid sending angry You-Messages which usually bruise relationships, we need first of all to identify the *primary* feelings that made us "act" angry. One needs to ask: "Am I feeling hurt, neglected, ignored, afraid, unappreciated, or what?" After we have identified our primary feeling, then we can communicate that feeling to the other person. Invariably, it will be an I-Message rather than a You-Message, as in our example in which it was the nurse who owned the problem: "I have a problem with your getting out of bed to have a smoke in the bathroom. I'm really afraid you'll fall or open up your incision, and I'll feel terrible and responsible."

When You-Messages Are Not So Risky

We are not suggesting that You-Messages be permanently dropped from your communication with patients. They should be avoided, however, whenever patients convey that they own a problem. They are much less risky when your relationship is "on task." Referring again to the Behavior Window, these You-Messages are less risky when the relationship is in the No Problem area and you are sure that neither you nor the patient owns a problem. Often both persons can be joking with each other and the relationship is felt to be more like a friendship—so secure that Roadblocks often get bounced off each other, as in the following situations in which nobody owns a problem.

1. *Physician*: Nurse tells me you had an uncomfortable night. (Smiling) What are you trying to do, make your doctor look bad? (INTERPRETING)

   Patient: I can see I get no sympathy from you. Next time I'll have you called at home in the middle of the night. (THREATENING)

2. *Nurse*: (Ready to give a shot) OK, roll over on your side and prepare for target practice. (ORDERING)

   Patient: Hope you got a sharp needle for a change. I'm beginning to think you get some sadistic pleasure from sticking me! (INTERPRETING)

3. *Patient*: One of the nurses told me you're a Boston Celtics fan. I hope you have better medical judgment than your judgment of basketball teams.

   Physician: Who is your favorite team? (QUESTIONING)

   Patient: The Lakers, of course.

   Physician: You're in worse shape than I thought. (RIDICULING)

4. *Physician*: You're going to have an EKG. Take your shirt and shoes and socks off and lie down. (ORDERING)

   Patient: What comes next?

   Physician: Lee will hook you up.

5. *Patient*: Do you have to shave my chest? The last time it took months before the hair grew back.

   Nurse: What kind of work are you in? (PROBING)

   Patient: I'm in construction.

   Nurse: Maybe you'll have to wear a T-shirt to work for a while. (GIVING A SOLUTION)

The *critical* time to avoid the You-Messages is when you get a message or a clue (verbal or nonverbal) that the patient is experiencing some sort of problem or there is evidence of trouble in the relationship itself. We will next describe and illustrate the communication skills that have proven to be effective in confronting patients when you own the problem.

THE THREE-PART CONFRONTIVE I-MESSAGE

Confrontive I-Messages are the most difficult to put into practice in the precise form that is required for them to influence others to change. When some behavior of a patient is unacceptable to you because it gives you a problem, your most effective assertive statement will be a Confrontive I-Message that has three components. Ideally you want your confrontive message to achieve three goals:

1. Get your needs met through a change in the patient's behavior
2. Preserve the patient's self-esteem
3. Maintain the strength of the relationship.

The three-part I-Message has a high probability of achieving these goals. Following is an explanation of each of the three components.

Nonblameful Description of the Behavior That Is Giving You a Problem

The purpose of specifying the unacceptable behavior is to make sure the patient knows exactly what behavior is giving you a problem. You'll want to avoid arousing any unnecessary resistance caused by blameful or critical messages.

- Avoid: When you thoughtlessly refuse to return my calls to you . . .
- Better: I have a problem when I don't hear from you after I call.

It is important to describe only the *behavior* of the other person—what you can see, hear, touch. Avoid *inferences* about what the patient's attitudes or motives may have been. In short, don't let this part of the message create unnecessary defensiveness or resistance, which you will then have to overcome to get your needs met. Avoid such messages as "When you are inconsiderate of other patients on the ward. . . . " Far better is this message: "I have a problem when your radio is on loud."

The Tangible and Concrete Effect on You

People don't usually change a specific behavior unless they are quite certain it has a concrete and tangible effect on another. So you need to make patients understand clearly how their behavior concretely impacts you—

how it deprives you or threatens to deprive you of getting your needs met. Avoid any statements that point the finger of blame and make the patient feel guilty; instead, realize that chances are the patient did not intend to interfere with your needs. The tangible effects of the behavior should be believable to the patient. He or she must believe that the behavior *really* causes, or is likely to cause, these effects. If effects are untrue or if they seem too far fetched *to the other*, the I-Message will usually fail. It doesn't matter how much *you* believe the effects—*you* are not the one to do the changing. Tangible effects are often hard to identify. It may help to specify the possible tangible effects on you in terms of (1) costs to you in time, extra work, or money; (2) time off task, interference with your pursuit of personal and professional goals; (3) obligations or cleanup tasks caused by a behavior that will prevent you from doing something important or pleasurable to you; (4) subtle losses, such as loss of satisfaction or approval of others, or feeling unsuccessful. Here is a Confrontive I-Message that clearly conveys a tangible effect: "I have a problem when your radio is on loud, because then I have to take time to go answer the complaints of patients who can't go to sleep."

Your Feelings

This is often the hard part. Our culture teaches us either to deny or to hide our feelings. So for most of us it sometimes feels scary to reveal our feelings. Nevertheless, this is the important ingredient that gives the strength and legitimacy to your message. Leave out the feeling, and the I-Message is only cold logic. However, clearly and honestly expressed, your emotions will enable the patient to understand you at a deeper, more personal level and become more willing to help you with the problem you own. Expressing the feeling allows the patient to see how much you need his help. If you withhold the feeling, he or she may feel justified in thinking that there's really not much reason to change.

Avoid the tricky second meaning of the phrase "I feel." That construction is so often interpreted as, "I have the opinion that. . . . " So avoid such messages as "I feel you let me down" or "I feel you didn't really do your job." Here is a better way to express your feelings: "I have a problem when your radio is on loud, because then I have to take time to go and answer the complaints of patients who can't go to sleep; and that makes me very irritated."

For an I-Message to be effective, the feelings expressed *must be true*. And the degree of strength (e.g., from mildly annoyed, through angry, to rageful) must be reasonably believable. Undershooting, especially, will weaken your impact. And making up strong or impressive feelings that are not your real ones will destroy your message's credibility.

When sending the I-Message, your affect, tone of voice, facial expression, and body language must match the degree and kind of feelings described by your words. Your I-Message must be *congruent*—that is, your *inner experience* and its *outer expression* must match. Congruence gives believability and impact to your message, and it is probably the single most important factor in making your I-Message successful.

After you have identified in your mind (1) a nonblameful description of the patient's behavior giving you the problem, (2) the effect of that behavior on you, and (3) your congruent feelings about the effect, then you need to combine them into a sentence or two and have the courage to send your three-part Confrontive I-Message to the other person.

Try to start out announcing your ownership of the problem with the attention-getter: "I have a problem." From then on, neither the order of the three elements nor elegant phrasing in the final I-Message is too critical. What *is* important, however, is your intention, which should be to share— truthfully and openly—how the patient's behavior affects you, both tangibly and emotionally. And then you stop to give the other the opportunity to take responsibility for modifying the specific unacceptable behavior in a way that meets your needs and also is acceptable to the patient.

If you think about it, a good Confrontive I-Message is really an appeal for help from the other person. Experience confirms that when we appeal for help, the other person will be much more motivated to respond positively. Also, because good I-Messages don't suggest or demand your solution, the responsibility is left with the person to come up with a solution of his or her own. I-Messages obviously are not a method for *controlling* another person but a way of *influencing* the person to assume responsibility for self-control—that is, to choose to change the behavior because it is causing another a problem. I-Messages do not attack the other person's self-esteem, because they are not You-Messages about the *other* person— they are I-Messages about *you*.

Following are examples of good three-part Confrontive I-Messages:

1. *Physician*: I have a problem when you don't notify our office that you can't show up for your appointment. I feel irritated, because we have missed the opportunity to give your time to another patient.

2. *Nurse*: I have a problem when you take so much time before letting me give you your shots. I worry that I won't have time to take care of all my other patients.

3. *Physician*: I have a problem when you don't get a Pro-time every three weeks, but let it go as long as five or six weeks. I really worry that you might have a stroke, and that would make me feel sad.

4. *Nurse*: It's a problem to me when you refuse to take your daily walk down the hall that Dr. Seward ordered. I'm afraid you're delaying the time when you can go home, and I might get blamed for it.

Dr. Naomi Remen, then at the Institute for the Study of Humanistic Medicine in San Francisco, reported a blood-drawing experience with children with cancer that illustrated how amazingly effective an open, honest, and direct I-Message confrontation can be.

One by one each child was brought in by the nurses. How I dreaded those mornings! The hour went by in a blur of fearful children, as I filled test tube after test tube, never confident that I would be able to "hit" the next child successfully.

One morning the door swung open and in marched a resolute five-year-old boy with a diagnosis of leukemia. He was followed by four nurses, one of whom said, "This is David." I was surprised to see so many nurses and was about to ask why, when one of them lifted David to the table. Suddenly there was a mass of struggling women: "Got his leg? I have his arm. Watch out, he bites . . . ," and the room was filled with David screaming and screaming.

I was appalled. Nothing in medical school had prepared me for this. I had never seen such a struggle. I later found out that this was David's ninth hospital admission, and that this identical ritual had been repeated countless times. I stood there ignored and shaken, as the nurses attempted to restrain the child. A little arm projected from under the white mound of their bodies. As it was smaller than the rest, I drew blood from it, assuming that it was David's. I said, "I have it," and one by one the nurses, wrinkled and sweating, got up, and left David alone and quiet on the table. He was watching me. My hands were shaking so badly that I could not transfer David's blood from the syringe into the test tube. I brought my hands up against my chest to steady the transfer. David said, "Why are your hands shaking?" All my training and conditioning could not have helped me to answer. I had many answers, ranging from "I didn't have breakfast yet," to "My hands are *not* shaking!"

Instead, I found myself saying, "I'm shaking because you yelled so loud you frightened me." I immediately sensed the strong disapproval of the nurses to my message and I was mortified. I had said the wrong thing—it had just slipped out. Later that morning I received a summons to the office of the Director of Nurses.

Did I realize what I had said? That I had revealed a weakness to a child whose only hope was his belief in our strength? I had damaged his trust in his doctors. I had behaved unprofessionally. The Chief of Service would be notified.

I had no response, but I did not apologize. Something kept me from apologizing. A few days later I was again in the treatment room at dawn. As I glanced anxiously over the list of patients, my eye caught David's name. I asked that he be called first, as I wanted to have it over with. The door swung open, and in walked David, followed by four nurses. But there all similarities ended. Waving the nurses back, he climbed up on the table and extended his arm to me. "There," he said, "I won't scare you this time." And he never "scared" me again. (Remen, 1975, p. 37)

One of a number of physicians who have been trained to be Parent Effectiveness Training (P.E.T.) instructors, Dr. Robert Daigneault, submitted the following two cases that clearly illustrate the effectiveness of Confrontive I-Messages (Daigneault, 1993):

Case One: Patient is a 20-year-old college student who came into the campus health center one afternoon just before closing. I saw him and diagnosed him as having a URI (cold). I recommended symptomatic treatment and he left the health center. The next day I learned that he returned after closing and had hassled the on-call nurse. He complained about the time he had waited to be seen, the brevity of the visit, and the fact that he had not been given a prescription. I was really annoyed by his behavior because I felt it was not warranted. I had no opportunity to do anything about it at that time, but within a month he came to see me again for another problem. After we had dealt with the reason for his present visit, the following conversation ensued:

Dr. D: John, I'm glad to have the opportunity to talk with you.

John: Okay, Doc, what's up?

Dr. D: Do you remember about a month ago, you came in with a cold and I saw you?

John: Yes, I do.

Dr. D: Well, I learned that you returned after I left and complained to the on-call nurse about how you'd been treated.

John: Did I? I don't really remember.

Dr. D: Well, I just wanted you to know I was annoyed by your complaining, since I had given you the opportunity to tell your concerns at that visit. (I-MESSAGE)

John: Sorry, Doc. I didn't think that what I did would bother anyone.

Dr. D: Okay. I just wanted you to be aware.

As you can see from this case, confrontation with I-Messages may be brief, and does not have to be elegant. Dr. D continued to serve as the student's primary physician. Thus, this confrontation did not in any way interfere with their further relationship.

Case Two: Sixteen-year-old female with diabetes. She had been diagnosed but was not checking her sugar levels or following her diet. She had been hospitalized on two occasions because of her failure to do the above.

Dr. D: Good morning, Carrie. I was just talking with your Mom about your diabetes. She's quite worried.

Carrie: She's always worrying. I'm doing okay.

Dr. D: I'm sorry, Carrie, but I have a problem with what you just said. (I-MESSAGE)

Carrie: What problem?

Dr. D: You said that you were doing okay. I disagree, and I'm concerned because you're not testing your sugar levels or following your diet, and that has resulted in two hospitalizations. If you are to stay out of the hospital, I need your cooperation. (I-MESSAGE)

By confronting Carrie, Dr. D gave Carrie the problem.

SHIFTING GEARS WITH ACTIVE LISTENING

Although I-Messages have proven to be the most effective way to influence another person to change unacceptable behavior, there will be times when even the best three-part I-Message will trigger such responses as these:

1. The patient may respond with guilt, remorse, or chagrin: "I'm so sorry" or "I didn't know. . . . "
2. The patient may get defensive: "Nobody told me" or "I'm working as fast as I can."
3. The patient may deny any responsibility: "I forgot," "I was much too busy," "Nobody told me."
4. The patient may respond by showing resistance to change and little concern for the sender's feelings: "It's what I need to do," "I don't really see a need to change."

Such responses tell you that your Confrontive I-Message caused the patient a problem—a lot of resistance to change or various strong feelings. Recall that Active Listening is the appropriate and effective skill when the patient owns the problem. So now that your I-Message gives the patient a problem, it's prudent to stop your assertive/confrontive posture (moving forward) and change to a listening/understanding posture (moving backward)—shifting gears to back off for the moment. Here are two examples.

1. *Nurse*:	I have a problem with your taking so much time before letting me administer your shots each time. I'm afraid I won't be able to get to my other patients. (I-MESSAGE)
Patient:	I really hate those shots. They hurt a lot, and I've always been a baby about pain.
Nurse:	You've always been afraid of pain, and these shots really hurt. (SHIFTING GEARS WITH ACTIVE LISTENING)
2. *Physician*:	I have a problem when you say you don't walk every day. I'm afraid the circulation in your legs will get worse, and that would make me feel I haven't done my job well. (I-MESSAGE)

Patient: It takes too much time. Right now I'm swamped with
               work at the office.

Physician: It sounds like your work has a higher priority right now,
              so there's no time for walking. (SHIFTING GEARS
              WITH ACTIVE LISTENING)

When you hear such responses to your Confrontive I-Messages, more often than not it is useless to keep hammering away with repeated assertive messages. Shifting gears, however, makes the other person realize that you understand where he or she is now and that you are not trying to get *your* needs met *at his or her expense.* In addition, you'll find that shifting gears with Active Listening—once or as often as necessary—very often will dissolve the patient's feelings or resistance. People find it much easier to change after they feel the other person understands and accepts how difficult their changing might seem to them.

You may find it necessary to repeat your original I-Message or send an even stronger one and shift gears again if you still get resistance to change or hear strong feelings. Or you may find that your best efforts fail to influence the other to change, leaving the relationship with a conflict to be resolved.

CHAPTER SUMMARY

Consultant–client relationships are most effective when both parties feel free to self-disclose—to share their feelings, needs, and problems. Studies have shown that self-disclosure in relationships is reciprocal—that is, when health professionals freely communicate their thoughts, feelings, and problems, their patients are encouraged to do the same. Self-disclosure is also a critical way to prevent problems in relationships. The most effective self-disclosure is in the form of an I-Message, which can be used by health professionals (1) to express their opinions or beliefs, (2) to prevent any problems occurring in the future, (3) to respond honestly to patients' requests or demands, and (4) to influence patients to change behavior that is causing a problem for the health professional.

A graphic model of relationships, called the Behavior Window, has proven to be useful in understanding (1) the concept of problem ownership; (2) the need to use different skills, depending on who in a relationship owns the problem; and (3) the importance of focusing on specified *behaviors* of patients rather than making speculative assumptions about their traits, intentions, or motives.

Confrontive I-Messages are effective ways to influence patients to change unacceptable behavior. However, they are *most* effective when the confrontation carries three components: (1) a description of the specific behavior that is causing the problem for the health professional, (2) the tangible undesirable effect it has, and (3) whatever feeling the health professional is experiencing. Such three-part Confrontive I-Messages also carry the least risk of hurting the relationship and the best chances of influencing patients to change.

On the other hand, high-risk confrontations are messages that point the finger of blame or evaluate the patient as a person. Such messages, called You-Messages, hurt relationships and generate resistance to change. Messages that convey the health professional's anger to patients are really disguised You-Messages, and they carry a high risk of generating resistance to change. However, identifying the primary or underlying feeling produced by a patient's behavior and then coding that in the form of an I-Message can greatly decrease the risk and increase the patient's willingness to change his or her behavior.

Even well-coded three-part Confrontive I-Messages sometimes will produce resistance as well as strong emotional reactions, in which case shifting to the all-purpose Active Listening skill will communicate acceptance of the patient's feelings, prevent hurting the relationship, and often bring about a willingness to modify behavior.

Dealing Effectively with Conflicts

A cooperative process leads to the defining of conflicting interests as
a mutual problem to be solved by collaborative effort. It facilitates the
recognition of the legitimacy of each other's interests and of the
necessity of searching for a solution that is responsive to the needs of
all.

—Morton Deutsch, *Distributive Justice*

In the previous chapter, we introduced I-Messages, the effective communication skill for making patients aware of the needs of health professionals.
There are four kinds of I-Messages:

1. *Declarative I-Messages*, which convey one's values and beliefs to
   another
2. *Responsive I-Messages*, which convey one's willingness or unwillingness to do what someone asks you to do
3. *Preventive I-Messages*, for influencing someone to do something
   in the future that will meet your needs
4. *Confrontive I-Messages*, for influencing someone to change a
   behavior that is depriving you of meeting some need.

Although these self-disclosing communication skills are effective ways to prevent or change specific patient behaviors that are unacceptable to health professionals, there will be times when even good I-Messages will fail to achieve their intended purpose, resulting in a conflict of needs between physician and patient. The focus in this chapter is on interpersonal conflicts and methods for resolving them.

The fact that conflicts can and do occur in relationships with patients is certainly not a new idea. Among medical practitioners who have contributed to the medical literature about conflicts in physician–patient relationships, Dr. Timothy Quill has written most persuasively about the need to negotiate such conflicts to meet the needs of both parties, stressing that sometimes barriers cannot be easily worked through and can interfere with the creation of a therapeutic alliance. He then lists six negotiation strategies needed to resolve conflicts in the physician–patient relationship:

Separate people from the problem

Clarify the conflict

Brainstorm about possible solutions

Focus on common interests, not positions

Use objective criteria where possible

Invent new solutions where both parties gain. (Quill, 1989, p. 54)

These strategies are quite similar to the conflict resolution system that we will describe and illustrate in this chapter. However, we first should examine the concept of conflict.

CONFLICTS IN RELATIONSHIPS

Ask people what words come to mind when they think of conflicts in their various relationships and you will hear words like the following:

dispute	battle
disagreement	struggle
quarrel	contest
argument	cross words
fight	hostility

come to blows	scuffle
oppose	collide

Most of these are "fightin' " words. They commonly suggest serious trouble, difficult problems, situations people prefer to avoid.

Much less common is perceiving conflict as a positive experience—a situation that can turn out to be rewarding. In fact, conflict has both perils and possibilities—both dangers and opportunities. The famous educator and psychologist John Dewey wrote that conflict stirs us to observation, invention, and creativity, the sine qua non of reflection and ingenuity. Conflict can also be perceived as the "gadfly of thought." It can bring about constructive evolutionary changes in relationships and organizations; it can promote more intimacy between persons; and it can actually make relationships more interesting and stimulating.

Conflicts are opportunities to identify problems that need to be solved and that, if not solved, would foster dissatisfaction, need deprivation, resentment, or anger. Unresolved conflicts can escalate into nasty fights in which persons see each other as adversaries, and they can bring about alienation from those whom one has previously respected, cared for, and loved.

Both the perils and the possibilities of conflict are certainly present in relationships between health professionals and patients. Physicians may come to dislike some patients; patients may fire their physician and look for another they hope they can get along with. Patients can also go to the extreme and file malpractice lawsuits against their physician. A survey of physicians who had been sued for malpractice found that almost two-thirds of them thought malpractice could be significantly reduced by improved communication (Shapiro et al., 1989).

If a relationship appears to have no conflicts, it often means that one person has power over the other and the weaker person is too fearful and submissive to raise potentially conflicting issues or has learned to give in and play the role of peacemaker in the relationship. However, in consensual and collaborative relationships, where there is no power differential, conflicts are much more likely to surface. Health professionals who choose to establish collaborative and cooperative relationships with patients will find it easier to create a climate in which conflict not only can come forth but also can be defined and resolved creatively, thus avoiding the perils of the win/lose and power-struggling posture of paternalistic or authoritarian relationships.

However, the traditional model of relationships between health professionals and patients has not been one of equals. Because health professionals are seen by patients as possessing the resources to solve their problems, patients feel more dependent on health professionals and thus are inclined to avoid conflict by not asserting their own needs. The head nurse in a large metropolitan hospital spoke of the power differentials in her relationships: "At work I feel powerful in relationship to patients as well as the nurses I supervise; and when any of them act up, I don't hesitate to show them who's boss. But at home, my husband runs the show, and I find myself submitting to his wishes in order to avoid arguments."

Like this head nurse, most people see conflict as ending up with someone winning and someone submitting. It is what we call "either-or thinking"—either I win and you lose, or you win and I lose. Fortunately, there is a third outcome—where both win or nobody loses. We will examine each of these three outcomes of interpersonal conflicts.

Method I: You Win, Other Loses

In this way of dealing with conflict, you use your power to try to get your needs met, but at the expense of the other suffering need deprivation. Those who win may get their way, but they will also get some unwanted reactions from the losers who are left with unmet needs.

They begin to fear you.

They criticize you behind your back.

They form alliances to counteract your power.

They start avoiding you.

They lie to you.

They tell you only what you want to hear.

They don't tell you all their problems.

Method II: You Lose, Other Wins

With this method of dealing with conflicts, the other person gets his or her needs met at the expense of your not getting yours met. Method II is commonly used by those who don't like conflict—they want peace at any price, so they give in. Now it's the one giving in who will have the unwanted reactions:

You'll feel resentment or anger.

You'll feel frustrated.

You'll start feeling depressed, apathetic.

You'll stop revealing your needs or problems.

You'll lose respect for yourself, develop low self-esteem.

You'll covertly meet your needs in other ways, in other relationships.

Method III: The No-Lose Method

This method requires a commitment from both persons not to use power to meet their needs at the expense of the other person not getting his or her needs met. Conflict is seen by each as a problem to be solved, requiring a mutual search for a solution that will be acceptable to both—a no-lose or win-win solution.

Most of us have learned from our experiences with parents and other authoritarian adults that conflicts are most commonly resolved by Method I or Method II. Consequently, changing to No-Lose Conflict Resolution is not easy, especially for those people who have gained a position of power in their relationships. However, making the commitment to find no-lose solutions to conflicts in a relationship can be very gratifying, bringing such benefits as these:

1. It allows conflicts to surface, be expressed, defined, and resolved with constructive and equitable solutions.

2. People learn that conflict can produce exciting and interesting changes; they start seeing conflict positively, as a signal that their relationship needs fixing in some way.

3. Each person takes personal responsibility for getting her or his needs met, but not at the expense of the other. (Unwillingness to lose is a key element.)

4. People are far more willing to deal with real conflicts, not just superficial ones.

5. The same conflict won't keep coming up over and over again when it is resolved fairly and amicably.

6. Better, and often more creative, solutions to conflicts are generated when all parties involved participate, thus benefiting from each person's creative thinking.

7. Both people are far more committed to carrying out the decision when they participate in making it rather than having it imposed on them—another application of the participation principle.

8. People feel closer to each other—resentment and hostility are replaced with warm feelings and closeness.

9. Both will see this as a model they can use to solve conflicts in other relationships.

Resolving conflicts so nobody loses is another application of the Six-Step Problem-Solving system described in Chapter 2. The six-step method has proven to increase the probability of finding a mutually acceptable solution to conflicts, whether between two people or two groups.

SETTING THE STAGE FOR NO-LOSE CONFLICT RESOLUTION

The first task, obviously, is to get both parties to the conflict to agree to drop all ideas of winning (or losing) and enter into the no-lose process. The reality is that many people have had no experience with this way of resolving conflict—at home, at school, at work. Consequently, the one person who is familiar with the method will need to influence the one who is not.

One way to do this is to send such Declarative and Preventive I-Messages as these:

I would like to see if we can sit down and together try to come up with a solution that would be acceptable to both of us.

I really want you to meet your needs. Let's see if we can come up with a solution that meets your needs and also meets mine.

I wouldn't want our relationship to end without our trying to find a solution that we both can accept and live with. Would you be willing to try?

It may be necessary to send strong Confrontive I-Messages, such as the following:

I get so frustrated when you seem unwilling to consider any solutions except your own, so I'm really disappointed at not being able to put our heads together to find a mutually acceptable solution.

I feel terrible when we have a disagreement and you seem to give in and give up. It makes me feel like I'm the winner and you're the loser. I would like us to try a new way of resolving our conflicts so that nobody loses.

Of course, you may also need to shift gears after such confrontations and do Active Listening to the other person's response to your I-Messages. Experience tells us that most people really don't like win-lose solutions or unresolved conflicts, so they'll usually welcome the opportunity to try a new method.

After reaching agreement to try the new method, both must understand each of the six steps. You may describe them or let the other person read them from some source. It is also important to agree on a definite time free of distractions, because No-Lose Conflict Resolutions can be time-consuming. With some conflicts you may want to use a chalkboard or chart pad, or simply paper and pencil.

THE SIX STEPS OF NO-LOSE CONFLICT RESOLUTION

Step 1: Define the Conflict in Terms of Needs, Not Solutions

Because most people have learned to see conflicts in terms of *competing solutions*, it is critical in Step 1 to define the conflict accurately in terms of each person's *needs* or *fears*:

What do I really need or want?

What fears do I want alleviated?

As an example, suppose a patient and her physician have a conflict about the treatment for her breast cancer. Rather than defining the problem in terms of competing solutions—surgery against no surgery, lumpectomy against mastectomy—physician and patient first should state their needs. The patient might fear losing her husband's sexual interest or might not want to be disfigured. The physician's need might to be avoid metastasis.

The importance of the distinction between needs and solutions seems to be supported in the article, cited earlier, by Emanuel and Emanuel

(1992). They emphasize that the ideal of shared decision making involves contributions from both physician and patient: patients bring their "aims and values" (what we call our needs or fears), after which risks and benefits of various treatment options can be evaluated, and physicians can then bring forth their expertise and preferences for available treatment alternatives.

In Step 1 it is of critical importance for the health professional to use Active Listening frequently, in order to demonstrate acceptance and understanding of the patient's needs and fears.

Step 2: Generating Alternative Solutions

In this step both health professional and patient generate alternative solutions or combinations of solutions (like lumpectomy plus radiation). This step should involve putting their heads together, trying to be creative, suspending judgment and evaluation so as not to impede the creative process. At the outset of Step 2, the health professional should suggest they adopt a ground rule of withholding evaluations of alternative solutions until the list has been completed.

Step 3: Evaluating the Alternative Solutions

Both health professional and patient now are free to evaluate the alternative solutions generated in Step 2. What are the pros and cons, the benefits and risks? What are the costs? What solutions meet the needs of both patient and practitioner? Does one solution seem more workable? Sometimes a brand-new solution will emerge, or an earlier one will be improved by a modification. Failure to test the solutions in Step 3 decreases the chance of ending up with the best decision.

Step 4: Deciding on a Mutually Acceptable Solution

Now a commitment to a mutually acceptable solution can be made. When all facts are out in the open and the various solutions have been weighed and analyzed, the parties will usually close in on one solution that satisfies both persons. Often it will be a combination of two or more of the suggested ideas. Pushing a solution on the other person or agreeing to a solution you don't like should be avoided. If both people don't freely choose the final solution, chances are it will not be carried out.

When you appear to be getting close to a solution acceptable to both, state that solution very clearly, to make certain both of you understand it. When you do, you may want to put the solution in writing to be sure that future misunderstandings can be verified against the decision that was made.

Step 5: Implementing the Solution

Decide *who* does *what* by *when*. An important assumption of No-Lose Conflict Resolution is that the participants are responsible and trustworthy, and that given support and understanding, they'll carry out their obligations. Monitoring and nagging tend to foster dependency and resentment rather than individual responsibility. However, because many people are unaccustomed to No-Lose Conflict Resolution, at first they may not assume full responsibility for carrying out solutions. If, as time passes, the other party to the decision fails to carry out his or her part of the agreement, you'll need to reopen your discussion with a Confrontive I-Message such as "I'm really disappointed and upset because we made an agreement about this conflict and you haven't stuck to it!" The other person then realizes that you expect him or her to be responsible.

Step 6: Evaluating the Results of the Solution

This step is often overlooked when resolving conflicts. Not infrequently a solution reached in Step 4 turns out to be inadequate. Circumstances may have changed, or you find weaknesses in the solution. Sometimes one or both parties find they overcommitted and agreed to something that was impossible to implement or didn't really meet their needs. Solutions obtained with No-Lose Conflict Resolution need not be seen as carved in stone. If at first you don't succeed, go back and search for another solution that works better.

A CASE STUDY

Following is a case study reported by Dr. Timothy Quill (1983), in which he and a patient worked out a mutually acceptable solution in the form of a contract that required certain compromises by both parties. The six steps of No-Lose Conflict Resolution are identified by the author (TG). Both physician and patient stated their specific needs clearly and yet arrived at a unique solution that wasn't expected by Dr. Quill. Fortunately, that solution enabled the relationship to last 11 months or more.

A 58-year-old insurance salesman received total disability for chronic pain. He had a 34-year history of pain dating back to shrapnel injury in World War II, and had had seven abdominal operations and a transurethral resection of the prostate three years ago complicated by sepsis and myocardial infarction. In the past year he had seen 30 doctors for left flank and low-back pain, almost all of whom he believed were incompetent. The patient had tried drugs, acupuncture, and self-hypnosis, but nothing worked. He was taking high doses of a narcotic analgesic and a tricyclic antidepressant, each helping a small amount. The narcotic was administered by his wife at his doctor's insistence. The patient's psychiatrist of 15 years said the pain was in his body, and prescribed the narcotic that his internists and urologists would not because of the risk of addiction. The patient was writing a book about the incompetence of the medical profession, and angrily queried if I would be any different.

After hearing the patient's history I had to ask myself the same question. I responded by agreeing that the patient had had some terrible medical experiences, but how could I be of help after the other doctors had failed? [DEFINING THE CONFLICT] The patient responded with two clear requests: he wanted to get his narcotic pain medicine without being called an addict; and he wanted surgery, a myelogram, or at least a cystoscopic to try to take the pain away. [PATIENT'S NEEDS]

Because I knew my limitations in each of these requests, I believed I could establish a relationship with this patient. My counter proposal had several components. I was willing to prescribe the narcotic without calling him an addict or questioning his need each time, provided he give the medicine to himself on a regular basis every four hours rather than as it was needed for pain, a more appropriate regimen for chronic pain. [PHYSICIAN'S NEED] After assuring myself that his condition was not dangerously acute, I told him that I would not intervene in any way until I had all of his records, and only then for clear medical indications. [POSSIBLE SOLUTION] I told him that if I were to be his primary physician, he could seek no further consultations, medical opinions, or medications without checking with me first. [POSSIBLE SOLUTION] I stipulated we would meet on a regular basis for 20 minutes whether or not he was having pain.

Only at that time would his medicine for pain be renewed or reviewed and this "non-symptom dependent visit" was to keep our relationship from reinforcing his pain. [POSSIBLE SOLUTION]

To my surprise, the patient agreed to the proposal. [MUTUALLY ACCEPTABLE SOLUTION] He tested our agreement once by returning in two weeks with worsening pain and microscopic hematuria, but again nothing was seen on examination and no new intervention was ordered. [EVALUATING THE SOLUTION] The patient's records were voluminous, and showed that he had had all appropriate diagnostic tests done at least twice, and that all his previous physicians found him to be a troublesome patient. The microscopic hematuria had been intermittent for several years, and had not yielded a diagnosis despite several complete urologic evaluations.

Our relationship is now 11 months old. We continue to meet monthly when I renew his prescription for the narcotic analgesic. [IMPLEMENTING THE SOLUTION] I have never questioned whether his pain is real, and continue to work with him in his struggle to live with it. I repeatedly reinforce the fact that his pains have been thoroughly evaluated, that no additional intervention is necessary at this time, and that I will keep an open mind to new medically treatable conditions that may arise in the future. [IMPLEMENTING THE SOLUTION] The patient has not sought other opinions and gets all his medicine, including his narcotics only from me. His previous requests for surgery or other procedures have diminished. [EVALUATION OF SOLUTION] (p. 232)

Dr. Quill concluded as follows:

This patient and I worked out a contract—a relatively complex one that has maintenance of the status quo as a major principle. I am not trying to take his pain away (doctors had been trying unsuccessfully to do that for 35 years), but rather to do no harm through unnecessary surgery and help him learn to live with his pain. I have made my limitations and expectations clear, but he is free to end our relationship and seek another physician if he wishes more aggressive treatment or is dissatisfied with the agreement about medications. The contract needed compromise on both our parts, but it also provides explicit guidelines about what we can expect from each other. These clearly negotiated operating principles have allowed us to control medical problems that at first glance seemed overwhelming and out of control. (Quill, 1983, p. 232)

By looking at conflict positively, one can perceive it as welcome evidence of unmet needs in a relationship rather than as a struggle to win. Conflict can be a healthy vehicle for open and honest communication, for recognizing deep feelings, for reaching new understandings. People grow from disagreements—learn from each other, change their beliefs or opinions. And relationships can become richer and stronger from working together to find solutions that allow both persons to get their needs met.

Another illustration of a successful No-Lose Conflict Resolution was described by Dr. Quill:

I will illustrate the strategy by the example of an anxious patient with irritable bowel syndrome who has been extensively tested and treated with no improvement in the diarrhea or cramping. Both doctor and patient are frustrated by her lack of progress, and this sense of frustration is preventing them from having meaningful, direct communication. The conflict has boiled down to a difference in opinion about the role of psychosocial problems in the illness, which the patient angrily and steadfastly denies. ("You'd be frustrated too if you had uncontrolled diarrhea.") The physician's strategy is to separate the people from the problem by suggesting that they are both frustrated by her persistent bowel problem (not by each other). He attempts to clarify the conflict by asking the patient to discuss her frustrations openly and fully and by doing so himself. In the process, the physician learns that the patient feels she is being accused of being a hypochondriac, and that she feels the physician is not taking the physical side of her ailment seriously enough. The physician openly expresses belief in the interaction between mind and body in this illness, and acknowledges that his frustration over the patient's unwillingness to explore the psychosocial dimensions of her illness may have led to a lack of emphasis on the physical symptoms. They establish a common interest of making the patient feel better and lessening her symptoms, but the physician acknowledges that many times this problem is life long, and helping the patient adjust to it rather than "curing" it may be the best he can offer. Such conversations where conflict is openly addressed and explored often facilitate the process of over-coming barriers, although many deep-seated barriers such as this can only be fully addressed over time in the context of a long-term, consistent doctor-patient relationship. (Quill, 1989, p. 55)

Making the No-Lose Conflict Resolution method work will require extensive use of both Active Listening and I-Messages, in addition to (1) showing respect for the needs of the patient, (2) trusting the patient's potential for creative thinking, (3) being open to ideas different from your own, (4) refusing to revert to Method I or Method II, and (5) being persistent.

The question most often asked by persons who have no experience with No-Lose Conflict Resolution is "What if you simply can't come up with a mutually acceptable solution?" True, stalemates may develop—sometimes because the parties did not follow the six steps, or one or both are still in a win-lose posture and a power-struggle frame of reference.

Here are some things that often work when a mutually acceptable solution is hard to come by.

1. Go back to Step 2 and generate more solutions.
2. Go back to Step 1 and try to redefine the conflict—there may be a hidden agenda.
3. Ask "What is impeding us? Why aren't we able to find a mutually acceptable solution?"
4. Ask "Do we need more data?"
5. Focus again on the *needs* of each party so that you get away from competing *solutions*.
6. If there are requirements for resolving the conflict within a particu-lar time period, make this clear to the patient.
7. Suggest you both "sleep on it" and resume problem-solving later.
8. Suggest trying out one of the solutions for a limited time period on an experimental basis.

THE HEALTH PROFESSIONAL'S AREA OF FREEDOM

If you think of No-Lose Conflict Resolution as a form of sharing the decision-making authority with the patient, it becomes obvious that health professionals can share no more decision-making authority than they already have. Some issues that come up in relationships with patients will be outside the professional's area of freedom, and therefore will be nonnegotiable.

Think of the square below as representing the total freedom of a health professional if there were absolutely no limits.

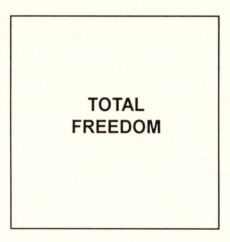

The figure below shows how the area of freedom of a health professional will be reduced by several factors.

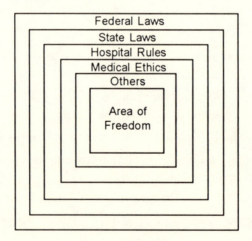

Most health professionals will have a greatly limited area of freedom, but one in which they can accept mutually determined solutions to conflicts with patients. What can they do if solutions are generated that fall outside their area of freedom? Here are some suggestions:

1. When a solution is proposed that is outside your area of freedom, tell the patient and explain why.
2. Active Listen to the disappointment or other feelings the patient expresses.
3. Invite ideas as to what might be other solutions acceptable to you.

WHEN AGREEMENTS ARE NOT HONORED

Although No-Lose Conflict Resolution generates much stronger motivation to carry out the agreed-upon solution, sometimes a patient may not honor the agreement. Do you then resort to Method I? Do you blame or reprimand the patient? Far better that you try less risky approaches:

1. Remind the patient of the agreement you both agreed to accept.
2. Use I-Messages to communicate how not honoring the agreement tangibly and concretely affects you negatively. Shift gears with Active Listening, if necessary.
3. Bring the issue back for additional problem-solving if the previous solution has been difficult for the patient to honor.

CHAPTER SUMMARY

Experiencing a conflict in person-to-person relationships conjures up "serious trouble," "emotional battles," and other frightening prospects. However, conflicts also bring possibilities and opportunities for constructive changes and more intimacy in relationships. In fact, in collaborative relationships conflicts are more likely to surface, as opposed to authoritarian or paternalistic relationships, where conflicts don't always get out in the open.

How conflicts finally get resolved is more critical to a relationship than *how many* conflicts arise. The ideal way to resolve conflicts is using a method in which the parties agree on a solution that meets both of their needs—no one loses. No-Lose Conflict Resolution involves six separate steps that, if followed, greatly increase the probability of a successful outcome.

Using both Active Listening and I-Messages helps the parties understand each other and reach a mutually acceptable solution. Suggestions were given as to what can be done when acceptable solutions are hard to reach, when agreements are not honored, and when a solution is outside the health professional's area of freedom.

Chapter 7

Helping Patients Cope with an Adverse Diagnosis

Thank you for letting me know by your voice and your expression that you cared when you told me the diagnosis.
—Patient with leukemia

In his book *I Don't Know What to Say* (1988), Dr. Robert Buckman tells the following story.

Ellen, a patient with cancer of the ovary . . . was a senior personnel officer. . . . Her doctor told me, "She will simply not allow me to tell her what is going on, and I am concerned that you may not be able to offer her treatment." . . . Her first words . . . were, "If it's cancer, I don't want you to tell me." . . . She told me of the . . . deaths of five members of her family suffering in a similar manner and thought that if she knew it was cancer, all the fight would go out of her. Without specifying the name of her disease, I described the treatment, its side effects and the various support services that we could offer. . . . She recognized the treatment as chemotherapy. When I confirmed that it was, she smiled . . . and said, "Oh, . . . I knew it was cancer anyway." From that moment on, she relaxed and tolerated the treatments . . . with considerable calm. (Buckman, 1988, p. 50)

What to tell the patient when a life-threatening diagnosis is confirmed? In the past, it was customary to keep the patient from discovering the diagnosis. "The patient would lose hope" was the normal excuse. "It would be too harmful for the patient to know" was another reason given. The patient's chart was off-limits to the patient and family. Part of this was because words like "cancer" were unacceptable in polite society. Even today, when the patient first hears the word "cancer" or "malignancy" from the doctor, shock sets in and he or she hears little else that is said that day. These words no longer seem prohibited by our culture. Still, there are families of patients who feel that the knowledge itself will hasten the end of life and rob the patient of the will to live. "The news alone will kill our mother," they say.

Following are some of the feelings shared by patients in regard to how they were told they had a life-threatening illness:

> When you told me over the phone that I had cancer, I felt devastated and wished you had told me in person, so I could see you cared.

> When you told me my husband had cancer, we were in a crowded, noisy hallway, and I felt the need of privacy, so I could cry and ask questions.

> I felt confused and irritated when you gave me a lot of details about my husband's tests before you told me he had cancer. It would have been better if you could have made it simpler and more direct.

> I liked it when you indicated you would stick with me, not abandon me if your curative therapy did not work.

> When you said you would continue to keep yourself informed about research and new therapies for my condition, I felt reassured.

Elisabeth Kübler-Ross (1969) describes her interaction with a patient who kept his feelings hidden until approached with an open-ended question:

> The staff was convinced that the patient did not know the great seriousness of his condition, since he never allowed anyone to get close to him. He never asked a question about it, and seemed in general rather feared by the staff. The nurses were ready to bet that he would never accept an invitation to discuss the matter with me. Anticipating difficulties, I approached him hesitantly and asked him simply, "How sick are you?" "I am full of cancer" was his answer. The problem with

him was that nobody ever asked a simple straightforward question. They mistook his grim look for a closed door; in fact, their own anxiety prevented them from finding out what he wanted to share so badly with another human being. (Kübler-Ross, 1969, p. 55)

The current legal doctrine of informed consent states that all patients must be informed of all the diagnostic and therapeutic options, plus the risks and imponderables of each choice. It may be difficult to inform the patient adequately if the diagnosis is very complicated or the patient is not capable of understanding. Some physicians have difficulties putting their recommendations in simple lay language that can be easily understood by non-medical people.

Sometimes the patient must know the seriousness of the situation in order to make important family decisions, such as who will be responsible for child care. In those cases the question for physicians becomes not "Shall we tell the patient?" but "How do we break the news most gently?" The goal is to be able to speak freely about the diagnosis without necessarily equating it with impending death. The door should be left open for hope—that all is not lost. The message that should be communicated to the patient is that it is a collaborative relationship of physician, family, and patient fighting together, no matter what the end result. If this is the message, the patient will not fear isolation, deceit, rejection. Most important, he or she will continue to have confidence in the doctor, understanding that everything that can be done will be done.

From a medical standpoint, keeping the patient uninformed is usually not helpful. A number of studies show that most patients with cancer want to know the diagnosis and the seriousness of the situation. Most want to know so they can make future plans. Other studies show that patients kept unaware of the diagnosis suffer more with depression, anxiety, and loneliness.

Is any harm done if the patient says he or she does not want to know? If the patient is relaxed and functions normally without knowing what is going on, then the facts need not be thrust on him or her by the physician or family or friends, especially if there are no medical or family reasons the patient should know. If the patient is saying "Don't tell me," but seems depressed or anxious, it sometimes helps to share the facts. The patient wants to ask the questions but is afraid of the answers. There is a conflict of needs to consider.

In our collaborative model of the physician–patient relationship, patients need to be told the complete medical situation if they are to participate actively in the treatment choices, especially if the diagnosis is AIDS or cancer. In fact, the current legal doctrine of informed consent states that all patients must be informed, not only during the first stage of illness or following confrontation, but also later from time to time. Consequently, the basic problem for physicians becomes using their interpersonal skills to encourage patients to talk about their *reactions* to unfavorable diagnoses.

Physicians, nurses, and family members have a difficult time when the patient has been told the diagnosis but has trouble accepting it. It may help health professionals and family members to be more sensitive to and accepting of patients' reactions to unfavorable diagnoses by understanding the findings of Elisabeth Kübler-Ross (1969) from her work with the dying. She found that patients often go through the following stages as they experience the progression of symptoms in a life-threatening illness:

Denial	Bargaining
Anger	Guilt
Fear	Acceptance
Depression	

At any of these steps, health professionals will find their communications skills invaluable. Patients who cope with shocking news by *denial* will invariably give verbal or nonverbal clues, which the physician or nurse can feedback with empathy and acceptance, keeping in mind that it is the patient who owns the problem. When people are in a denial mode, Active Listening often facilitates their moving into a deeper and more basic problem, which usually is more solvable.

Recent studies have revealed much about anger as a coping mechanism. As described in Chapter 6, anger, a response we manufacture is often a secondary feeling following a more basic feeling—such as fear, embarrassment, loss of control. Anger itself is directed outward as a You-Message to another person or to a situation in one's environment. Active Listening helps people get beyond the anger, identify the primary feeling, and begin dealing with what is really bothering them. This process is apparent in the following case study.

David was angry at everyone around him. One month ago he was told he had Lou Gehrig's disease, which is uniformly fatal, with progressive loss of strength in the muscles of the body. He was a professor in the law school at age 45 and had just been promoted to a new and challenging position. He was told there was no treatment and that most individuals lived about 18 months after diagnosis. David, who had always been a calm, easygoing person, began to viciously attack those around him. He yelled at his son for not making top grades as a law student. He screamed at his wife, bringing up an affair he believed she had had 20 years earlier. He was irritable at work, and his colleagues began to shun him. All this occurred while he was still relatively unimpaired and able to get around fairly well. The author (WSE) was asked by a friend of David's to see him. The conversation went as follows:

D: My son is getting lazy and not working like he should, and this is irritating to me.

WSE: You feel angry at your son's not working hard.

D: I've told him he must get top grades if he wants a good appointment when he graduates, yet he ignores my advice.

WSE: You feel he is not listening to your advice, and this is irritating.

D: Everyone seems to be doing irritating things. My wife was unfaithful 20 years ago, and the memory of that episode drives me wild. I can't get it out of my mind.

WSE: That painful memory sticks with you.

D: Even those lawyers at the school expect me to do their work and mine, too. It's not like it used to be when I was their age.

WSE: At work you feel others are not doing their share of the work.

D: A year ago things were so different and peaceful. Why are these people now driving me crazy?

WSE: Something has happened in the last year that has taken away your peace of mind.

D: Yeah. It's this damn illness that really is unfair. And why now, just as I start a new position? Why didn't it wait till I retired? Till I had completed my career?

WSE: This illness makes you mad—it came much too early.

D: Yes. Why didn't this happen to old Jacob C—who retired from his law firm 10 years ago and is bored with life. I've got so much I want to do—I haven't got time to be sick and possibly die.

WSE: Doesn't seem right to have this happen when you've so much to do—very irritating. Why shouldn't it happen to people who have nearly finished life?

D: It makes me so mad. I feel like kicking everyone I see, especially those healthy people around me.

WSE: You are angry with those healthy people for being well when you can't be.

D: That's what's so irritating. I have no control.

WSE: You feel at the mercy of fate, and that's really bothering you.

D: I think I've been taking my feelings out on my family and friends. No wonder they seem to be avoiding me.

Several such conversations with David helped him get more in touch with the causes of his anger, and he was then able to let up on those around him. As is apparent, Active Listening was used almost exclusively, and the Roadblocks were avoided. Consequently David realized he was feeling a lack of control.

When life is threatened, probably the most frequent feeling is loss of control. Most of us like to have decision-making power over events that affect us, and when we don't, we feel very angry or frustrated. Illness, loss of job, and an accident are examples of loss of control that lead to anger. Whom do we curse? God? Fate? Luck? We take it out on those closest to us—our spouses, families, friends, nurses, doctors. Those who are recipients tend to take this anger personally and to return mad for mad. This exacerbates the situation and often leads to explosion.

This case history illustrates the use of Active Listening to help patients see that their primary feelings were about loss of control. Individuals who have been most in control in their jobs, their families, their businesses commonly have the most trouble accepting being dependent on spouses or on the medical team in the hospital when they develop a serious illness. Being told what to do, what to wear, when to sleep and wake, makes patients angry, especially when some of the orders are given by nurses' aides—because they are far down the intellectual scale (in the view of these patients) or because they are women.

One of the most difficult problems to face, but a fairly frequent one, is how to manage conflict between patient and spouse, or patient and another close relative. The author (WSE) has found that No-Lose Conflict Resolution and a lot of Active Listening by both parties can be very effective in helping participants find a mutually acceptable solution.

Sometimes the patient and spouse relate to each other with repeated critical statements and judgmental You-Messages that keep the relationship stirred up and angry. Active Listening can be very helpful in producing peace. A training program called Relationship Enhancement (Guerney, 1982) teaches spouses to listen to each other and reflect back the feelings each has heard being expressed by the other. Some call this "pencil talk" because the speaker holds a pencil (or any other lightweight article) in his/her hand while expressing feelings about the other, and does not relinquish the pencil until the other can use Active Listening to reflect those feelings accurately. The other then holds the pencil while describing feelings. It is gratifying that a better understanding frequently results from using these skills when conflict breaks out.

A first step in teaching this process is to reflect back to each speaker in turn the feelings being expressed. Such a dialogue is illustrated in the following paragraphs.

Wesley, a 73-year-old man had a diagnosis of ALS (Lou Gehrig's disease) six–eight months before. The disease had advanced to the point where he was wheelchair dependent. Someone had to push the wheelchair because he was unable to turn the wheels. He had to be helped to the bathroom, to be placed on the toilet, to be moved from wheelchair to bed, and even to be turned over in bed. He could feed himself and swallow, but his voice was becoming affected and his speech slurred. On a visit, the following dialogue occurred. His wife, Meg, usually participated in our conversation.

WSE: How has it been for you two since my last visit?

Meg: I'm afraid I blew up yesterday and unloaded on Wesley. I told him how angry it makes me that he won't cheer up and find some pleasure in whatever time he has left. He won't enjoy the nice weather, or the friends who call or visit. He has lost his sense of humor, which used to be one of his nicest characteristics.

WSE: You feel irritation at Wesley when he won't try to get some enjoyment out of life.

Wes: I hate being dependent on everyone, not being able to take care of myself, and I don't enjoy sitting all day in this wheelchair. I feel discouraged, nothing seems funny or amusing. I would love to feel different, but I don't know how.

WSE: You find it hard to find enjoyment when you can't do anything for yourself.

Meg: I cook up the most delicious dishes, and he eats them without any enthusiasm. That makes me frustrated and mad.

WSE: You feel irritation when he won't enjoy your cooking.

Wes: I have lost all my sense of smell or taste, and her best cooking is the same as chewing rags to me.

WSE: It's hard to be enthusiastic when everything tastes the same.

Meg: I wish he would act enthusiastic sometimes, even if he doesn't feel it.

WSE: You would like him to fake it now and then.

Meg: Yes, but when I say that, I realize it is my feelings or frustration I'm worried about, not his.

WSE: You realize you're wanting him to change his attitude so you'll feel better.

Meg: I guess I'm tired and discouraged, and have hoped he would change so these feelings would be lessened.

This conversation and several others like it seemed to help Meg tolerate her frustrations better, and as she became less judgmental of Wesley, he became less irritable and regained some of his wry humor. However, these two people never did learn to Active Listen to each other without a third person present. Couples who do not respond to these techniques apparently have communicated with each other this way for so long that they have no desire to change. Reflecting back to each other, as was done with Wesley and Meg, can be helpful. Then one may ask if they would like to learn to Active Listen to each other. Unless there is an affirmative answer, one has no alternative but to continue Active Listening to both.

There is also a common expectation that the medical profession should be able to cure anything and everything these days, so when people are told there is no treatment or that their bodies are no longer responding to maximum treatment, anger results. It is common to expect medicine to cure any illness or replace any part, just as we expect a mechanic to repair our automobile. And if the illness becomes a huge financial drain, as is often the case, anger is intensified.

To counteract this common feeling of loss of control, physicians, nurses, caregivers, and family members need to utilize the participation principle, described in Chapter 2, in order to give patients as much control as possible over their environment—encouraging them to make decisions about when to schedule their baths, wearing their own pajamas, making menu selections, and other such choices.

When a life-threatening illness is diagnosed, another coping response can be fear. Fear is many-sided and varies tremendously in degree. First there are fears of physical pain as a disease progresses, and fear of loss of ability to get around independently. I (WSE) experienced this kind of fear when I had a bloody bowel movement 15 years ago. I immediately suspected cancer of the colon and had horrible visions of having a colostomy and becoming dependent as well as losing dignity and bowel control. It proved to be a benign colon polyp that was easily removed, but the fear was genuine. I was surprised to learn that I had less fear of death than of the disabilities and indignities that I might experience.

There are also fears of losing loved ones, fears of leaving family unsupported either physically or financially, fears of an unpleasant afterlife, fears that conflicts will not be resolved before death. For men there is often the fear of being afraid, not appearing courageous, not acknowledging this painful emotion.

Again, what can caregivers, either professional or family, do to help alleviate these fears? First, look at fear as a clue that the *patient owns a problem*. Thus, Active Listening is the skill of choice to help patients share their feelings and have them accepted by a sensitive listener.

In the following case history, Active Listening brought about a tremendous change in attitude:

Andrew, a patient referred from doctors at the Veterans Administration hospital, had been going downhill physically for two and a half years with a generalized malignancy. In spite of continuous chemotherapy, he had gone from 230 to 100 pounds. He had once been a powerful man and a strong patriarchal figure for his children and for his wife, who was now caring for him at home. An open-ended question served as an invitation for Andrew to self-disclose.

WSE: Andrew, how do you feel about what's happening to you now?

A: I don't like it, but I have to live one day at a time. Can't let it get me down.

WSE: You don't like losing weight and strength, but you need to be brave about it.

A: I'm doing all the doctors tell me to do, but I wish I knew something else I could try.

WSE: You would like to find some way to control what's happening to you.

A: All my life I took care of myself, with nobody's help. If I wanted something, I could work hard and get it. It makes me mad that I can't overcome this illness on my own.

WSE: You're discouraged that you can't use your strength and will to get well.

A: I haven't told my family, but I've been silently praying that God will help me get well. It scares me that the answer from God seems to be no, and I remember sins I have committed along the way. Am I going to hell? That really scares me. Maybe I don't deserve to go to heaven.

WSE: It's scary to pray and not have your prayers answered the way you had hoped, and you're scared you're going to die and not go to heaven.

A: I'm glad I told you that. I feel better. Maybe I should tell my wife. She knows something is going on that is making me worry more.

Andrew continued to share his fears and anxieties, and his depression became less deep. The last months of his life were much more peaceful.

Caregivers and family members need to be alert to the physical signs that indicate *depression*: loss of appetite, loss of interest in surroundings, no interest in the daily news or local events, insomnia (waking in the middle of the night), flat facial expression with disappearance of smiling. It is important for family or friends to alert the physician to these symptoms because the patient will frequently deny them. Depression is one of the hardest concerns to deal with, because depressed patients don't feel like talking, and initiating a dialogue is often difficult. Depressed patients may want to be alone, to avoid human contact. This phase is often very discouraging for caregivers; they often resent the emotional unresponsiveness of patients and equate their lack of response with ingratitude. It is hard to fix tasty meals for a spouse who has no appetite and refuses to eat.

Both professional and family caregivers can try to enrich a patient's environment by getting him or her to play cards or listen to music. It has been found to be stimulating to give at-home patients chores as a way to prevent the feeling of helplessness.

Depression may be so severe that it is relieved only by electroshock therapy. Electroshock therapy currently is considered much safer and less destructive to brain tissue than it was a few years ago. There may be slight memory loss, but it is not severe and doesn't reduce the person's lucidity.

Depression waxes and wanes, and sometimes alternates with periods of high hopes and optimism, with no obvious explanation for the transition.

Another response to illness is *bargaining*. Patients try to make deals between themselves and their doctors, or with God. "Doctor, I'll accept your recommendation for further chemotherapy if you'll promise it will cure me," or "I'll buy the church that new organ if you, God, will let me get well." One of the most frequent bargains patients make is for time. "God, I'll be willing to go peacefully if you will let me live through my daughter's wedding next month." Later comes "But, God, don't forget, I've got another daughter." These bargains are seldom kept. It is helpful for caregivers to accept these efforts to bargain for what they are—messages that communicate patients' efforts to develop some hope where there has been despair.

Empathic Active Listening again is the best choice of response, although open and honest Responsive I-Messages may be appropriate when patients demand things—for example, "I wish I could promise you a speedy recovery, but I can't honestly do that."

Serious illness can cause patients to feel that they are being punished for some "sin." This may be especially true for AIDS patients. Can a caregiver or family member reduce this feeling of guilt? Reassuring the patient with "You've nothing to feel guilty about" is a commonly used Communication Roadblock that seldom will erase the guilt. However, it will help to demonstrate by Active Listening that the patient's feelings are accepted as normal and natural. Active Listening will encourage the patient to talk freely about these guilt feelings, as shown above in the case of Andrew, who was suffering from guilt and fear of punishment before and after death. Active Listening also brought about a change in the guilt feelings of Laura, a 40-year-old woman with a husband and three teenage children when she developed lung cancer. Laura had been a heavy smoker since age 12 and was suffering guilt for causing her own cancer.

L: Why, oh, why, didn't I listen to my parents when they tried to get me to stop smoking?

WSE: You're feeling remorse that you didn't stop smoking when your parents advised you.

L: Right. Now I feel as though I caused this terrible illness that may shorten my life—and what did I get out of it?

WSE: The enjoyment of years of smoking now doesn't seem worth it.

L: I'm punishing my husband and my children, who are having to care for me and will have to grow up without me if I don't make it.

WSE: You feel like you're punishing them by requiring them to care for you and then lose you.

L: I feel ashamed of my addiction. I'm a weak person—even bad.

WSE: You feel that you're weak and bad for smoking.

L: When I hear myself say that, I know it's not true. I've been a good wife and parent.

WSE: You realize you're not really "bad" because you've been a good wife and mother.

L: I made a mistake, but I was not bad. And this is not some kind of punishment. I've given love and support to my family and friends.

WSE: Maybe they don't feel punished by giving you love and support when you need it.

Laura's guilt continued to bother her but was greatly reduced in intensity. Her death was peaceful.

To help the patient accept an unfavorable diagnosis, Active Listening is an invaluable skill for encouraging ventilation of painful feelings. When patients experience these feelings being *heard and accepted* by a caregiver, they often gain deep relief.

Chapter 8

Special Problems Dealing with AIDS Patients

The true physician has a Shakespearean breadth of interest in the wise and the foolish, the proud and the humble, the stoic hero and the whining rouge. He cares for people.
—Tinsley Harrison, *Principles of Internal Medicine*

Jonathan, a 28-year-old computer programmer, was a good athlete, playing tennis, squash, and volleyball, before he developed AIDS. He had a well-proportioned body of which he was very proud. When he first developed Kaposi's Sarcoma, the hard, brownish and pink spots on his arms or legs were easy to conceal with long-sleeved shirts and long pants. His hair began to fall out due to his chemotherapy treatment. He became very depressed over his self-image and what his friends must think of his appearance. One day on his visit to Doctor Cathcart, the infectious disease specialist who was caring for him, the following conversation took place.

Jon: Doctor, I'm looking terrible. Isn't there something I can do to keep these spots from spreading to my face and hands?

C: Your appearance is really bothering you.

Jon: Yes. I used to be a good-looking guy, but now I'm a mess. I can see my friends recoil when they see me with my hair falling out.

C: You can see a look of shock when they look at you.

Jon: I may be imagining about my friends, but I feel shocked when I look in the mirror.

C: You may be projecting your own discomfort onto your friends.

Jon: Yes, that may be it. They don't seem to be paying attention to how I look. But I'm worried that the Kaposi's Sarcoma is not responding to the chemotherapy yet. I'm still having the nausea, weight loss, and hair loss that goes with it.

C: I agree. The lesions are no longer responding to our most powerful chemotherapy. How would you feel about stopping the chemo?

Jon: That would feel like we're both giving up and might be very depressing.

C: There is a new experimental drug that is just becoming available. The bad news is that its side effects are even worse than what we've been using.

Jon: Well, I think I'll go off all drugs now and concentrate on healing the relationships with my parents and my uncles and aunts.

C: That is certainly a reasonable decision, and I'd be glad to work with you on that basis.

Jonathan stopped his drugs, his chemotherapy symptoms improved, but his skin lesions continued to grow. He got a rousing cheer from members of his support group when he showed up in shorts and a short-sleeved shirt. "To hell with what people think," he said, "I'm going to be comfortable on these hot days."

This brief interaction between Jonathan and his physician illustrates the sometimes incredible effectiveness of a few moments of empathic listening to patients with a life-threatening disease.

A major epidemic in the last decade of the 20th century is the rapidly increasing prevalence of acquired immune deficiency syndrome (AIDS). AIDS, which at this time is invariably fatal, is caused by the HIV virus. This agent destroys the immune system, without which humans are susceptible to a host of infections and malignancies that eventually cause death. There are several characteristics of AIDS that make caring for people with this disease more stressful emotionally than caring for patients with other life-threatening illnesses.

The first stress for caregivers or family members is their own risk of infection with the HIV virus. There is no danger of infection if one does not come in contact with the blood or tissue fluids of the patient. Blood transfusions from a certified blood bank are now considered safe, but there remains a very small risk (1 in 6 million transfusions) because rare donors are so recently infected that their serum does not yet test positive for the HIV virus. The major routes for the transmission of infection are still unprotected sex and the use of unsterile needles by intravenous drug users. Professionals caring for HIV-positive patients are at risk from accidental needle sticks and lacerations from broken glass syringes and similar injuries. The risk is small, and can be reduced further by using universal precautions (masks, gloves, protective goggles) during all invasive procedures on all patients, since there is no way to know if the new or emergency patient is HIV positive. Studies of health care workers with parenteral (below the skin) exposures when caring for AIDS patients has estimated an infection rate of 0.4% (Gerberding et al., 1990) and even lower rates with mucosal exposure (mouth, nose, eye) (Gerberding et al., 1987). In the case of an accidental exposure when caring for an HIV-positive patient, antiviral drugs are often given quickly, in the as yet unproven hope that infection may be prevented.

AIDS patients frequently cause problems for caregivers, as is shown by this exchange between Roger and his nurse.

Roger, age 23, was an intravenous drug user who sometimes traded used needles and syringes with friends. His nurse at the clinic found out about this after Roger had become HIV positive. She realized that this was causing her to own a problem, and she remembered it called for a Confrontive I-Message.

Nurse: Roger, when you exchange needles with others, it upsets me because it is quite likely your friends may become infected, if they are not already.

Roger: I realize that may cause a problem for my friends, but I can't seem to get off IV drugs and I don't know where to get sterile needles.

Nurse: I recognize your difficulty. Our clinic can provide you with a supply of fresh, clean needles. I'll help you arrange for them.

Other emotional issues that serve as barriers to the care of AIDS patients are anger at noncompliant drug users; fear that AIDS patients in the waiting room may scare other patients away; concern over the complexity and rapidly changing state of the art in therapies for AIDS (a very rational fear!); discomfort when talking about sexuality and safer sex practices. Caregivers need to recognize these areas of discomfort and seek people or groups with whom they can openly discuss these feelings.

Despite this low rate of transmission to health care workers, a high level of fear persists that may not reflect the actual risk of becoming infected (Cook, 1990). In 1987 half the physicians surveyed believed they had a right to refuse care to a patient with AIDS, and 15% said they would actually refuse to care for them (Merrill et al., 1989). More recent studies of senior medical students and nursing students showed that this fear (Meisenhelder and LaCharite, 1989) was the principal cause for their avoiding AIDS patients. Thorough education and conscientious use of safety precautions has reduced the fear of contamination on the part of caregivers. Reduction of this fear allows a less stressful, more empathic relationship to develop.

The second factor that makes caregiving tension-filled for both professionals and family is the fact that AIDS at this time is uniformly fatal. Cancer patients' care may sometimes be depressing, but there are many cancer cures and long-term survivors. Burnout rates are high among physicians and nurses who treat AIDS patients almost exclusively. Frequent short periods of time off or sabbaticals from dying patients seem to be helpful in reducing burnout. Support groups for caregivers where feelings can be ventilated may also be useful and healing.

Nurse Nancy Thomas had worked in the medical intensive care unit for several months without respite. This unit was almost exclusively dedicated to the treatment of AIDS patients, and there was an average of one or two deaths a week; usually they were young males in their twenties or thirties.

Nancy became irritable and impatient, which was not at all like her usual outgoing, optimistic personality. Cynthia R., the unit supervisor, effectively used her confrontive skills and Active Listening in dealing with this problem.

CR: Nancy, when you spoke harshly to Joe Suddeth just now, I was surprised and somewhat concerned. (I-MESSAGE)

NT: Joe made me feel exasperated because he won't take his pills.

CR: You felt irritation when he wouldn't comply with your treatment. (ACTIVE LISTENING, SHIFTING GEARS)

NT: He's rapidly getting worse, and I can't stand many more deaths on this ward.

CR: Yes, there has certainly been a rash of deaths lately.

NT: And they've mostly been young men, even just boys in some cases. They're dying in the prime of life.

CR: All these deaths of young people are depressing you.

NT: Cynthia, I like the work here and I feel it's fulfilling. But I need some time off, I guess, to recover a bit.

CR: We have two new nurses coming in a week. You can take a month off when they start.

NT: Thanks. In the meantime, maybe I'll go to that caregivers support group you told me about.

Sometimes hospice workers who are treating AIDS patients with comfort care only find they own the problem produced by a patient.

Hospice Nurse: Jacob, I'm upset and fearful since I found the full bottle of pain pills hidden in your bedside drawer. (I-MESSAGE)

Jacob: I've been collecting them for weeks so I can end my discomfort if it gets too bad.

nurse: I understand you want to have some control over your situation if the pain gets intolerable. (SWITCHING GEARS TO ACTIVE LISTENING)

Jacob: Yes. I've made peace with my parents and sisters, and I see no sense in suffering several more months with this pain.

Nurse: I'm sorry I can't leave these pills in your dresser. I'll talk to Dr. Jones when he comes in and ask him to talk to you. He is very good about listening to the patients with problems and feelings like yours, and perhaps he can help. He sometimes is willing to increase the dosage of pain medication to levels that relieve the pain although it may shorten life.

The third factor that can make AIDS care more stressful than care for patients with other life-threatening illnesses is the homophobia that exists in society and among many health professionals. Since this disease was first (and continues to be) manifested in homosexual males, many physicians and friends find themselves feeling anger, revulsion, and hostility toward patients when the diagnosis is AIDS. This interferes greatly with the development of an empathic relationship with the patient.

A study of third- and fourth-year medical students' attitudes toward homosexuals and AIDS patients was significant. This study of University of Mississippi students (Kelly et al., 1987) indicated that students viewed homosexual patients (regardless of their illness) in a highly negative way. In addition, AIDS patients (relative to leukemia patients) were seen as much more responsible for their disease, deserving of what happened to them, dangerous to others, deserving to die, deserving to lose their jobs, deserving to be quarantined. These were severely nonempathic attitudes that would significantly interfere with medical care. A comparative study of medical students at Columbia University College of Physicians and Surgeons (McCrory et al., 1990) showed much less negative attitudes toward homosexuals and AIDS patients, possibly because of the urban setting, where exposure to homosexuals was more common and less judgmental. The New York students had a more hostile attitude toward intravenous drug users.

The ultimate in judgmental homophobia was reported by Solomon (1990).

John, 36, had been hospitalized after he presented with severe signs suggestive of AIDS. A physician was assigned to his case and ran an extensive battery of tests to determine diagnosis. Confidence in the diagnosis of AIDS was increased when John developed *Pneumocystis carinii* pneumonia, a frequent complication of this disease.

John had revealed his gayness to his physician and had expressed his concern about the possibility of having AIDS. Upon relaying the diagnosis, the physician told John that his disease was a punishment from God, that his life was in God's hands, and presented him with a Bible. On subsequent visits the physician questioned John about his Bible readings and would berate him when he discovered that John had not been following his Bible study recommendations.

John, distressed by his physician's recommendations, spoke to a friend, who contacted the local AIDS caregiving group. John was advised of his right to change physicians and was given the name of a physician who was more supportive of gay men. The transfer was made and John died peacefully two months later, surrounded by friends and supportive caregivers.

Can homophobic caregivers or family members become respectful and empathic in dealing with gay men or women, and if so, how can this change be brought about? Studies show that it can be done.

Bauman and Hale (1985) at the University of Arizona developed a seminar for first-year medical students where half the class discussed societal biases toward homosexuals and the other half discussed nutrition.

The societal biases discussion group met with articulate homosexual men and women. Both groups took an attitudinal questionnaire before and after the seminars. The societal biases group became more accepting of the homosexual lifestyle; the nutrition group showed no change. The societal biases group students felt very positive about their experience and believed they could take better care of homosexual patients. Another study by Goldman (1987) showed the same thing.

Nevertheless, there are widespread beliefs that are barriers to dealing with homosexual patients. Most of the fear, anger, and hostility felt by the majority of individuals in our society, including many professional caregivers, is aggravated by the belief that sexual orientation is a choice that each individual makes. Some religious groups believe strongly that homosexuality is a sin and is so described in the Bible. However, psychiatrists and behavioral scientists are becoming increasingly convinced that homosexuality is not a choice. They have had no success in treating or reversing the orientation of gay men or lesbians. Siblings and parents often are certain that sexual orientation is present from birth. One mother says she can't imagine why anyone would choose to go through the misery of growing up gay, as her son did. Neuroscientists at the Salk Institute for Biological Science (LeVay, 1991) found one area of the brain smaller in gay men than in heterosexual men. Their colleagues at the University of California, Los Angeles (Allen and Gorski, 1992), found another area of the brain that is larger in homosexual men than in heterosexuals. These researchers believe the findings suggest that differences in sexuality are linked to differences in the structure of the brain—that homosexuality could be no more a choice than skin color.

Most gay males and many lesbians hate their orientation when it is first realized. They become homophobic themselves, their anxiety is increased, self-esteem is reduced. They often fear friends and family will reject them, that they will have future occupational difficulties, and that being gay or lesbian will not allow them to have children or families—it would have been so much easier if they had been born straight.

During this period of sexual identification, teenagers often develop deep and intense guilt or shame, overwhelming loneliness, inability to focus on school or work. Suicidal ideation, occurring in 40% (Jay and Young, 1979) of the gay and lesbian population, often appears at this time. Also, alcoholism often begins (Kus, 1988). Empathic, nonjudgmental caregivers who deal with adolescents are badly needed. The following dialogue in a nonmedical setting shows how facilitating Active Listening can be.

Tom was a high school junior whose grades had fallen from their previous high level. He had stopped participating in school affairs, including his favorite activity, the debating team. He skipped classes, appeared depressed. One of his teachers persuaded Tom to make an appointment with the school counselor, Mrs. Alford.

A: Tom, some of your teachers are worried about you. Your grades have dropped, and you've missed some classes.

Tom: That stuff we're studying is not interesting. It's boring.

A: You're finding it no longer interesting, and it's hard to focus on it. But you seem to have lost interest in the debating club also, and you were heavily involved in that.

Tom: I don't like some of the boys in that club.

A: Your relationship with some of the boys is not good.

Tom: I don't like being around them.

A: They are being unfriendly to you, is that it?

Tom: (hesitantly) Well, not exactly. They just make me uncomfortable.

A: How do you relate to the girls on the debate team?

Tom: They're OK—but I don't have much to do with them.

A: You feel relaxed with them but not at all close.

Tom: That's right. I don't want to have dates with them like the other guys, but I don't know why.

A: Who would you say is your best friend?

Tom: Donald, a senior, has asked me to go to a couple of concerts with him.

A: You enjoyed listening to music and being with Donald.

Tom: But it worried me when he put his arm around me in the car on the way home.

A: That moment of closeness disturbed you.

Tom: It felt good that he liked me, but I wondered if he was gay.

A: You had mixed feelings about his behavior.

Tom: It was even more worrisome when he kissed me on the mouth as he was leaving after the next concert.

A: You became more concerned the next time when he kissed you.

Tom: What worried me even more was I found myself kissing him back. I got to worrying, am I gay, too?

A: You're very concerned about your orientation toward boys.

Tom: Man, am I scared! If I'm gay, my parents and aunts and uncles will kill me. They hate gays and lesbians and think they're evil.

A: You're really frightened.

Tom: Yeah. But for gosh sakes, don't tell anyone what I've told you.

A: Certainly not. It's completely confidential, between just you and me. How are you feeling at this point?

Tom: Much better. Can we talk again?

Tom visited Mrs. Alford on a weekly basis for several months. With her assistance, primarily by using Active Listening, he was able to become more comfortable with his sexual orientation and to work through his self-esteem problems to some extent. His grades improved, and he began to debate again. He continued to keep his feeling secret from his family and acquaintances.

More and more gays and lesbians are beginning to identify and seek out physicians and other medical caregivers who can be accepting and empathic. In the past many gay men and lesbians preferred to "pass" as heterosexuals as long as possible, to avoid the rejection they feared from family and friends, and especially from employers. Living such a double life is often so stressful that it leads to a long-distance move, frequently to a large city where a new lifestyle can be adopted anonymously. Some who stay in their original environment find the stresses lead to alcoholism, suicide, drug addiction. Recently, however, contracting AIDS has served to bring many gay males out of the closet, whereas before they would have pursued long and successful careers without their homosexuality being known to any but their closest friends. This has been most notable among male movie and entertainment personalities. This notoriety may be very painful and aggravate the severe physical symptoms of AIDS. On the other hand, the gay community is beginning to demand acceptance, such as permission to serve in the military and to legally join in marriage.

Sometimes caregivers "own" problems created by the family of the patient with AIDS.

Cecil (pastoral counselor): I hear you're angry at your son, Rob, since he got AIDS and you discovered he is gay. I'm sorry you feel that way, because I've gotten to know and respect him in the last two weeks since he's been in the hospital.

John (Rob's father): Why shouldn't I be angry at him for being gay and choosing that disgusting lifestyle?

Cecil: You are unhappy he made the wrong choice.

John: Yes. He could have chosen to be heterosexual, like my other son.

Cecil: I've had long talks with Rob about his adolescence and the anxieties and struggles he had when he began to realize he had a different sexual orientation. He came to believe he really didn't have a choice.

John: We never talked about it, and perhaps I should have. I've always thought he was a fine boy.

Cecil: You must have strong feelings for him still, with that early relationship.

John: I guess I do.

Cecil: I know he desperately misses you and wants your acceptance. He knows he is going to die in the next few weeks or months.

John: Maybe we should get together and try to mend fences.

Cecil set up a meeting between Rob and John. They later told Cecil they both had a good cry together and regained an intimacy they had lost. Rob died after two months, with his father and brother at his side. Cecil's empathic listening greatly facilitated the reconciliation.

It has been found to be very helpful for gay men and lesbians with AIDS to select a close friend or lover and give that person a durable power of attorney for health decisions. If this is not carefully documented, the patient's family has legal rights in decision making if the patient becomes mentally incompetent. This can be unfortunate if the relationship between patient and family of origin is one of hostility and rejection.

Caregivers and family members can be helped by learning more about homosexuality, its facts, and its myths. They can attend workshops and discussion groups which help them identify their own biases. If a physician or nurse finds a strong degree of homophobia in himself or herself, it is better to recognize it and either change it or not accept referrals of gays or lesbians with AIDS or other serious illnesses. Homophobia is hard to hide from a sensitive homosexual individual.

Many of these special problems in dealing with patients with AIDS can be handled effectively if caregivers can stay informed about self-protection, can seek emotional support to deal with their inevitable stresses, and can recognize and deal with any homophobic biases that may prevent them from using nonjudgmental, accepting, and empathic skills with their patients.

One fortunate side effect of the AIDS epidemic is that the rapid change in treatments has resulted in a closer partnership between physician and patient than ever before. The new drugs are often experimental and patients know as much as physicians about them, so they work together more closely.

Chapter 9

Helping Patients Maintain Hope

I would like you to give me some hope along with the bad news, even
if the hope is small.

—Cancer patient

As mentioned in a previous chapter, most physicians now have become
convinced that patients usually want and need to know the diagnosis, and
some want to know the prognosis. Physicians know the *average* life span
after diagnosis of many progressive illnesses. Unfortunately, these figures
often ignore the exceptional patients who live far beyond the average, as
described by Bernie Siegel (1986). This may put physicians in a double
bind. How can they help patients maintain hope when they also feel
compelled to give them the probability statistics that have been accumulated
over the years?

There is increasing evidence that an attitude of optimism and hope can
improve physical symptoms and sometimes prolong life. For this reason, it
is imperative for physicians, nurses, caregivers, and family to be optimistic
and to promote a spirit of hope.

Some of the studies that support the idea that positive attitudes affect the
physical aspects of illness are quoted below. In fact, a new field of research
and treatment called psychoneuroimmunology is being developed, and
from it some additional statistical findings have emerged.

Dr. George Solomon and associates (1987) at UCLA Medical School studied six AIDS patients who lived far longer than expected and had been able to function at far above the usual level for this illness. Their findings suggest that positive attitudes and an optimistic personality were accompanied by a higher level of the positive components of the immune system that may help to offset the harmful effects of the loss of helper-T cells—a loss typical in AIDS patients. Another study by the same group found that positive attitudes, emotional strength, and attention to one's self-care, such as healthy diet and exercise, were correlated with relatively good immune measures, including what might represent compensatory increases in some categories of immune cells. Emotional distress, on the other hand, was accompanied by negative measures of immune functioning in people with AIDS. Some individuals infected with human immunodeficiency virus (HIV) have rapidly deteriorating immune systems; others do not. Preliminary studies suggest that HIV-infected men who are depressed show immune changes that favor the development of AIDS.

A Stanford University study (Bloom and Spiegel, 1989) reported that women with breast cancer who attended support groups lived an average of 18 months longer than women who had the same advanced degree of malignancy and were treated in similar ways but without support. Optimism was found to be a better predictor than pessimism of survival in men eight years after a heart attack (Ruderman et al., 1984). It was also better than the usual predictors, such as degree of artery blockage, quantity of heart muscle damage, level of cholesterol, or blood pressure. Only 6 of 25 of the most optimistic men had died, compared with 21 of 25 of the more pessimistic men.

Consider that patients with life-threatening illness hope for a number of different futures: (1) a physical cure; (2) a slow progression of disease, so they live as long as possible; (3) controllable pain; (4) minimal disability or loss of independence; and/or (5) friends, family, and physicians who will not abandon them as illness progresses. How can a person with a life-threatening illness gain and maintain such hopes, and how can caregivers support that optimism?

Attending physicians can do much to influence the prevailing patient attitude by careful attention to their own attitudes about the prognosis. If the physician gives up and says to the patient, "There is nothing more I can do," this will often throw the patient into despair. Many patients do not want their physicians to stop trying to find a treatment that will prolong life or produce remission of the illness. However, if the physician were completely open, honest, and direct in his or her disclosure, this I-Message to the patient would express *all* his or her feelings and knowledge. Using the five different components of the patient's hope, which we enumerated above, here are some Declarative I-Messages a physician might send (the numbers correspond to the numbers of the five components of a patient's hope):

> I'm sorry to say this, but as of now I don't know of any physical cure for the illness we have agreed you have. (1)
>
> I want to give you some statistics showing how long others have lived with this same disease. (2)
>
> However, I know that some patients have lived far beyond these averages. A few have even overcome this disease. (2)
>
> I want to tell you some of the things you can do that might prolong your life. (2)
>
> I also want to tell you how we can control the pain if that is a problem. (3)
>
> I would like to work with you to help you do a lot of things yourself, so you won't be so dependent on others. (4)
>
> I want to promise you that I will not abandon you, and I'll do what I can to influence your family to promise the same. (5)

To try to change a patient's attitudes by such Roadblocks as directing, advising, and reassuring usually conveys lack of acceptance and inhibits self-disclosure. It is important to emphasize again that the patient's attitude—optimism or pessimism, hope or depression—is a problem *he or she owns*; it is not the caregiver's or family member's problem. Consequently the patient can best be supported by empathic Active Listening.

Take the following example of dialogue between Virginia Josephs and Doctor Young.

> *VJ*: When you tell me I have several areas of cancer spread, it leaves me devastated and scared.
>
> *Dr. Y*: You feel scared and pretty pessimistic about it.
>
> *VJ*: I'm going to die, and that is very depressing.
>
> *Dr. Y*: You're really feeling like you're not going to recover.
>
> *VJ*: That's right, but I'm surprised at how much it helps to say it out loud.

Dr. Y: You find talking about it gives you some relief.

VJ: Yes. Admitting what I feel lets me accept that reality and move on to what I need to do with the time I have left.

Alice Ray was visiting her physician after a recent chest X ray and mammogram. It had now been two years after surgery for breast cancer, at which time she had no positive auxiliary lymph nodes. The following dialogue took place.

Dr. D: Mrs. Ray, the chest X ray was normal, your lungs were clear, and no sign of tumor. However, the mammogram shows a small lump in your opposite breast that is worrisome.

AR: My goodness, Doctor, what do you think it is?

Dr. D: There is no way to be sure what it is without another biopsy, but it could possibly be another malignancy.

AR: Oh, Doctor, I can't go through another major operation with all the pain and deformity involved. I just can't!

Dr. D: You hate to think about going through another operation.

AR: You have seen my chest now . . . all scarred up.

Dr. D: More scarring would be hard for you to take.

AR: But what would happen to me if I have another cancer?

Dr. D: I'm quite optimistic at this point. Besides, we could do a lumpectomy to make the diagnosis and treat the area with radiation if it is malignant. That would cause very little deformity and would adequately treat the tumor.

Alice Ray responded to her physician's empathy, as well as his optimism, and she underwent the treatment he prescribed with a good long-term result.

If the illness continues to progress and remission does not occur, patients still have hope that their physicians or family will not abandon them, that their pain will be controlled, that their last days will be peaceful, and that their good-byes will be comfortable and complete. Evidence that the health professional understands these hopes and will see that they are accomplished can be very helpful. An example of this was the case of John Shilling.

John Shilling had an esophageal cancer removed one year earlier, and had been doing well until one month before, when he lost his appetite and began to lose weight. Ultrasound and CT scans showed several areas of metastasis to his liver. The following dialogue occurred when he met with his physician.

Dr. S: John, the tumor has returned to invade your liver in several areas. This is why you have no appetite and have lost some weight.

JS: I was afraid that's what was happening. What can I do now?

Dr. S: We have found your kind of tumor doesn't respond to radiation therapy, so we will have to think of something else.

JS: It will take some time to sell my business, so I will need to live as long as I can. How long do I have?

Dr. S: That's impossible to say. People who have a strong desire to live seem to do better than passive people. You impress me as a fighter. How about looking at the therapeutic options that might slow down the progress of this tumor. (CONSULTING—USING THE PARTICIPATION PRINCIPLE)

JS: Let's do that.

Dr. S: There are two kinds of chemotherapy we could try. The first is very powerful and has a better chance of effectively slowing the tumor growth. Unfortunately, this drug causes uncomfortable side effects that would make active living difficult a good part of the time. The second drug has fewer side effects but is not as good at slowing the tumor.

JS: I need to be very active for at least a month to straighten out my affairs, so I'm tempted to take neither one, since you say that there is no chance of a cure.

Dr. S: You want to be able to function optimally for the present. You're right, these drugs would make you less effective.

JS: Will you continue to care for me if I'm not taking any medicine?

Dr. S: You bet. I'll see you as often as necessary, and we'll continue to confront this problem together.

JS: That's a relief. There is one thing I would like to ask you about, but I'm a little embarrassed to mention it, since it might be out of the realm of traditional medicine.

Dr. S: I'd be interested to know what you have in mind.

JS: A fried of mine had cancer a few years ago and felt he got considerable help from a cancer support group that practiced visualization of the immune cells attacking and destroying cancer cells. He felt this extended his life quite a bit. Would you have any objection if I tried it?

Dr. S: Quite honesty, I have no experience with visualization, but I would be interested to see if it proved helpful. Do you know how to contact such a group?

JS: Yes. My friend gave me the name of the contact person. I appreciate your support.

Dr. S was empathic, honest, and informative without taking away all hope. He did not promise a cure, but he did promise not to abandon JS and was supportive of his interest in trying nontraditional methods that were unlikely to have any negative side effects. He realized that JS needed to pursue this as a way to maintain some hope and control.

To provide the greatest support for a patient's hopes and beliefs, caregivers and family members should be hopeful themselves, believing that remissions of illness are always possible, and that as long as there is a desire on the patient's part to try new things, this will be encouraged.

Norman Cousins, the editor of the *Saturday Review*, recovered from a life-threatening illness for which there was no recognized therapy. He attributed his recovery to taking control of his attitudes and to a strong will to live. He described them in *Anatomy of an Illness* (1979). In a later book, *Head First, the Biology of Hope* (1989), he writes that the most insistent and critical questions put to him, generally by his physicians after the publication of *Anatomy of an Illness*, ran along these lines:

Aren't you afraid that the account of your experiences in combating illness will create false hopes in people confronting similar serious challenges? What about patients who try to apply cheerfulness, good humor, and a strong will to live—but whose underlying condition doesn't admit recovery or even improvement? Isn't life difficult enough for such patients without adding a burden of guilt? (Cousins, 1989, p.105)

Cousins answers these questions as follows:

People tell me not to offer hope unless I know hope to be real, but I don't have the power not to respond to an outstretched hand. I don't know enough to say that hope can't be real. I'm not sure anyone knows enough to deny hope. I have seen too many cases in the last ten years when death predictions were delivered from high professional station only to be gloriously refuted by patients having less to do with tangible biology than with the human spirit, admittedly a vague term but one that may well be the greatest force of all within the human arsenal. (Cousins, 1989, p. 104)

Bernie Siegel has also been criticized for creating false hopes by saying things such as this to his patients: "One out of ten patients with cancer of your type and stage will be alive 5 years from now. Why shouldn't you be the one?" Siegel's reply to his critics is that they are using false no-hope and that this is far more devastating.

Quoting Cousins again:

If the question about giving hope to catastrophically ill patients has validity, should it not also apply to hope connected to medical and surgical treatment? Since people reach out for medical care in hope of recovery, will they feel guilty if their bodies fail to respond to the physician's treatment? Is a physician justified in withholding such treatment because the hopes of the patient may exceed the realities of the case? The answer, of course, is that nothing should be held back that offers a chance, however remote, of improvement or prolongation even if complete recovery seems impossible. This applies not just to medical or surgical help but to psychological and spiritual care. Since there are imponderables that elude scientific predictions, the patient is entitled to a full mobilization of resources, including his own. (1989, p. 105)

A number of people have made the distinction between *curing* and *healing*, but none as eloquently as Sandra McCollum, herself a patient, when she gave a talk to a class of medical students. She stressed that the outcome of healing occurs "as a result of communication and caring in the relationship between the patient and physician." She believes that it is "the *disease* that separates patients from physician," and the distance becomes wider if patients hope or expect to be *cured.*

Ms. McCollum had been hospitalized over 50 times in the past 40 years, including two dozen times on a respirator for life support from 2 to 10 days. She recalls the exact words of her physician that communicated caring and healing:

Is there anything you need?
Think about what you want for dinner.

You'll have to tell me if the book you're reading is any good.
Is there anything else you want to tell me?

Sandra McCollum's final words to those medical students were these:

In spite of the difficulties, medicine truly is the noblest profession. In
no other career can you do so much to alleviate suffering and encourage the human spirit to soar. Each of you is a shining treasure—a gem
that is different in brilliance from every other. Over the years you will
cure much through your knowledge and skill. And each one of you
will heal your patients by *who* you are, just as surely as by what you
do.

Optimism, hope, the will to live—all these are proving important in the
outcomes of illnesses of all kinds.

Chapter 10

Helping Patients Find Meaning

> The belief has long died that suffering here on earth will be rewarded in heaven. Suffering has lost its meaning.
> —Elisabeth Kübler-Ross, *On Death and Dying*

When a chronic, progressive, or life-threatening illness develops, individuals may abandon all other interests and survival may become their only concern—the only meaning to their existence. How can caregivers and family members honor and accept this overpowering goal but at the same time help the patient find new meaning or fulfillment in the remaining months or years of life?

Some people find meaning by themselves and some do not, as suggested in the two following case histories.

Katherine was hospitalized for pain relief while she received her last tolerable radiation therapy for breast cancer that had spread to her spine. After she was taught by a nurse to regulate her own morphine drip, she asked for a wheelchair. When this was provided, she got herself into it with minimal help and began a daily routine of visits to many of the other patients with serious illnesses on her floor. She encouraged them to talk, she listened to what they said, how they felt, whom they missed. She smiled with some, cried with others. The patients looked forward to her visits, and Katherine was progressively able to reduce the amount of pain medication she required.

John was a patient on the same floor, but at a different time from Katherine. He was receiving chemotherapy for non-Hodgkins lymphoma. There were days he felt nauseated after a treatment, and he was losing some of his remaining hair (he was semi-bald already). He was visibly depressed, irritable, and angry. His nurses hated to go into his room, he was so hostile. His family members visited for only short times and at increasing intervals of time for the same reason. The hospital staff heaved a sigh at his discharge.

Both these people were dying of malignancies, but Katherine was able to find some fulfillment in the time she had left, whereas John approached his final weeks or months as meaningless, changeless fate. Neither could change the outcome, but Katherine chose to live fully until she died. She found meaning for herself and for those she visited.

Is there a way the physicians, nurses, or family members could have worked with John to overcome the anger, the hurt, the isolation he must have felt? Could someone have helped John by using Active Listening, by showing interest in him as a person?

Victor Frankl (1959) believes that a positive view of life results from an awareness that life has meaning under all circumstances and that each person has the capacity to discover meaning. Individuals can rise above ill health and the misfortunes of fate if they can see meaning in their existence.

According to Frankl "meaning" occurs at two different levels: ultimate meaning and meaning of the moment.

Ultimate meaning. The meaning of life is the awareness that there is order in the universe and each of us is a part of it. The religious individual will see this as divine law; a scientist will see order in the laws of biology, physics, evolution; a humanist will see meaning in ethics, morality, the laws of nature. Ultimate meaning can never be proved, attained, or understood. It is a matter of faith, of assumption, and of personal experience. Individuals can choose to live as though they are part of a purposeful, caring universal network or as though life is chaotic, unplanned, and hostile. No one of us living creatures will reach full understanding of the ultimate purpose of life; that will always be just over the horizon. But it is helpful in achieving a positive approach to life to believe that there is a useful purpose connecting our existence with the rest of the universe.

Meaning of the moment. Frankl's second level of meaning can be attained by everyone. In fact, to reach a level of fulfilled existence, this level must be reached. Frankl believes that each of us is a unique individual who travels through life in a series of different situations, each of which offers a meaning to be fulfilled—a chance to act in a meaningful way. Meaning can be found through what we do, what we experience, the attitude we adopt in situations of unavoidable tragedy. Finding meaning in the moment enables us to be a yea-sayer in the face of tragedy and to find meaning in meaningless situations.

Caregivers and family members can help patients find meaning by invitations to talk, open-ended questions, and a lot of Active Listening.

An individual who is a believer in a positive ultimate meaning, in either a religious or a secular context, will be more able to find contemporary meaning in a seemingly hopeless period because there is a built-in compass that points toward meaning. If one is not aware of ultimate meaning, one will do the best one can to find meaning for today's unique adventure or catastrophe.

In the past, most people found meaning in following the values supported by their culture or their religion, but that is changing. Children often reject parental values, church members resist the mandates of their churches, women resist the limitations of a primarily male society. Ethnic groups support different, sometimes opposite values. If traditional values are rejected, they must be replaced, or chaos results. Values and personal meaning are not moralistic rules but prescriptions for health. The consequence of seeking meaning in beliefs and behaviors that are not fulfilling may be mental or physical illness, depression, or suicide. It is not difficult to recall the names of many who did not find meaning in being rich or famous and finally ended their unfulfilled lives.

But how can caregivers help patients find meaning in the moment, especially in the presence of a life-threatening illness? Or, if you are the spouse or friend of a dying person, what can you do? Frankl's answer—that you can facilitate the patient's self-disclosure as he or she searches for meaning—is nothing new in religion or philosophy. It is new in medicine, where conscience is disregarded, and in psychiatry, where it is generally considered the result of parental and societal influences from outside the individual (the superego). Conscience is undoubtedly influenced by society and is highly personal, but each of us has an inner voice with the freedom to reject societal values.

Life is a roller-coaster. There are periods of frightening and depressing downs as well as ups filled with satisfaction and excitement, and plateaus of peace in between. There will be situations we can't change (fate) and experiences we can change (freedom); and, as the Serenity Prayer says, we must ask for "the wisdom to know the difference." Those who approach life with a "yes" are those who can find meaning even in the negative, unchangeable experiences of life. Even negative events such as wars and serious illnesses can give meaning to otherwise boring or meaningless lives. Wars stimulate patriotic fervor and excitement that can give new meaning to everyday existence. Illness may motivate sick individuals to take a new look at what is important in life and to initiate a search for added fulfillment.

Even those situations that are changeless allow us some freedom. Although we may not be able to change fateful facts such as permanent disability or approaching death, we always have the freedom to change our attitude toward these facts. And Active Listening can produce dramatic changes in attitudes toward a situation that is unchangeable. Death, loss of a limb, incurable disease, the restrictions of old age—these must be accepted, or the struggle to change the unchangeable will only weaken us. Here an empathic chaplain, social worker, friend, or caregiver can facilitate a patient's problem-solving process by Active Listening or helping the patient go through the six-step problem-solving process.

It is not always easy to distinguish between a situation that can be changed and one that cannot. In many personal, family, or job situations it is not clear whether meaning lies in fighting the problem or in accepting it. An individual with a progressive illness may find meaning in different attitudes toward the situation at different times, as identified by Elisabeth Kübler-Ross in the different stages that patients go through.

The major goal in being an effective helper of someone with an illness is to care about that person unconditionally—not using the communication Roadblocks that convey unacceptance and pressure to change—no matter what attitude or meaning he or she adopts. At the same time the helper must try to facilitate the patient's understanding that he or she can find meaning and purpose in the life span that remains. It is an interesting paradox that when people are accepted uncritically the way they are, they are more likely to explore ways to change. It is important that they know they have choices, even if they can't be cured of the illness. As the illness advances, there are still opportunities for fulfillment, as was illustrated by Katherine at the beginning of this chapter.

If the patient is interested and willing to seek meaning in the moment, one can help by inviting self-disclosure and discussion that may lead to the patient's finding a behavior that is fulfilling, not just something that provides pleasure, power, or money. Pleasure is a by-product of having done something meaningful; money and power are merely means to an end, not final goals. The patient might benefit in the search for meaning by talking about what meaningful goals might be possible if there were sufficient time or facilities.

There are a number of ways to help patients find their own meaning in the current situation. One way is by asking carefully considered, open-ended questions that suggest the areas in which meaning is most likely to be found. Some of the areas are described below.

SELF-DISCOVERY

The more patients can discover about their real selves behind the masks they wear for self-protection, the more real meaning they may discover. Since childhood people have leaned to put on masks so that they will be loved, accepted, successful. They have followed the advice of parents, teachers, peers, admired or beloved persons that allow them to be accepted or even to survive. An open-ended question such as "Which of your activities and behaviors are truly yours, as opposed to those that may be roles you play or masks you wear?" may stimulate personal insights. People can discover, when they are responding to a situation, if they are reacting (sometimes without being aware of it) to a meaning learned from parents, peers, or other important persons. And every time they have a glimpse of their *true* selves, they also have a glimpse of meaning. The self they can discover is not merely the self that has developed in the past but also the self that pulls them toward their goals.

There are more direct ways one can help patients discover themselves. The I-Message "I would like to know the real you" may at first bring forth a superficial answer, such as "I'm a salesman" or "Dorothy's husband," but Active Listening often brings deeper and more meaningful insights, such as "I am really a shy, anxious person." An open-ended question such as "What does your sales job mean to you?" may also lead to deeper self-discovery.

Another more direct approach to self-discovery starts with having the patient list the adjectives that describe how he or she sees himself or herself. Which of these describe things he or she likes about himself or herself? What does he or she dislike? Which of the negative traits would he or she like to change?

Indirect approaches to helping others know themselves are asking them to recall childhood memories, favorite stories, special experiences. "Why are those important to you?" "Did they have meaning?" Suggesting that patients make crayon drawings of themselves and asking, "Is this how you would like to be seen?" is a technique that has been used.

MEANING IN CHOICES

The second area in which caregivers, friends, and spouses can help patients find meaning is in choices. Choices are always available in any situation, but often patients are not aware of that fact. If they do not see choices, they feel trapped in a meaningless world. If people can see choices, they no longer feel helpless and therefore can usually find meaning. Active Listening can help patients distinguish situations they can change from those they must accept. The meaning in a situation that can be changed is to change it. Even in an unchangeable situation there is a choice: individuals can change their *attitudes* toward such situations. A person dying of cancer can lie in bed depressed or choose to live each of his or her final days admiring the scenery or sharing intimately with his or her family. The choices is always ours, and this certainly applies to the choice of attitude.

Do individuals with incurable illness have no choices? Can they find no meaning in life's remainder? Victor Frankl writes of his life in a Nazi concentration camp:

Do the prisoners' reactions to the singular world of the concentration camp prove that man cannot escape the influence of his surroundings? Does man have no choice of action in the fact of such circumstances? The experiences of camp life show that man does have a choice of action. There were enough examples, often of a heroic nature, which proved the apathy could be overcome, irritability suppressed. Man can preserve a vestige of spiritual freedom, of independence of mind even in such terrible conditions of psychic and physical stress. We who lived in concentration camps can remember the men who walked through the huts comforting others, giving away their last piece of bread. They may have been few in number, but they offer sufficient proof that everything can be taken from a man but one thing: the last of the human freedoms—to choose one's attitude in any given set of circumstances, to choose one's own way. . . . It is this spiritual freedom—which cannot be taken away—that makes life meaningful and purposeful. (Frankl, 1959, p. 86)

We all have choices—if about nothing else, then about our attitude toward life.

My work (WSE) doing one-on-one counseling has demonstrated that patients and their spouses or family members can work together to find new meaning in life for each other in the situation of life-threatening illnesses.

Individuals with recent onset of cancer, heart disease, progressive neurological illnesses have sensed that they can find new fulfillment by taking a
long and deep look at things in which they have sought meaning. It is
important for both professionals and friends to encourage the patient with
an open-ended question such as "Have you ever thought about what really
turns you on?"

UNIQUENESS

A job where you feel easily replaceable by another person or machine
will not seem as meaningful to you as one where you feel unique. Your
uniqueness may be expressed not so much by who you are as by how
important you are in relation to other people or situations. None of us, of
course, is completely irreplaceable, but there are circumstances when it does
make a difference whether we exist. Creative hobbies such as painting,
woodwork, weaving are satisfying ways to express uniqueness.

An 80-year-old man in a retirement home sat all day staring out the
window, seldom speaking, showing little interest in life. An artist
volunteered to teach painting to the retirees, and the octogenarian,
after some arguing, agreed to give it a try. He proved to have a unique
talent that the teacher encouraged. In a few months he was producing
excellent works. The teacher took a special interest and spent a lot of
time talking with the elderly gentleman. His mental alertness improved in parallel with his interest and involvement; his energy level
greatly increased. After a year, his teacher arranged a one-person show
of his work at a local gallery. He visited a clothing store to purchase
a suit for himself for the show and insisted that the clothing clerk
guarantee that this special suit would last at least 10 years. The
artist/teacher helped him discover a unique talent that gave a new
meaning to his life. As his interest developed, his attitude changed.

When a serious illness strikes, caregivers can be tremendously helpful
to patients by using open-ended questions for inviting and encouraging
them to seriously examine their life, their work, their relationships, especially from the viewpoint of unfulfilled dreams, talents, and interactions.
Can patients justify to themselves taking more leisure time for golf, bridge,
travel, reading? For those who reach the age of retirement, these are
legitimate leisure pastimes, but unless they express something unique about
the individual, they will not be fulfilling in the long run. The emphasis in

meaningful leisure is not on the activity but on the meaning and uniqueness that may be found in relationships with other people while fishing, playing golf, or playing bridge. One can help by using the helping skills that have proven to be so effective in getting patients to question themselves and discover the contribution each can make.

SELF-TRANSCENDENCE

This is the ability to reach beyond yourself and act for the sake of a cause that means something to you. It is perhaps the most fulfilling area in which we can find meaning, but it may be the most difficult to achieve. How can people who have learned they have a chronic or progressive illness feel wiling to do things for others when life has dealt them such an unkind blow? Who is going to feel like visiting other sick people when he or she has recently been diagnosed with advanced lung cancer, which is essentially incurable?

How can caregivers (doctors, nurses, spouses, friends) help patients recognize the value of helping others and become motivated to use this approach to finding meaning? One hopes the patient has already realized that giving love is the surest way to receive love. It is important not to overtly give advice or use other communication Roadblocks that carry the message that the patient's current attitude is not acceptable and should be changed.

One helpful technique is to act as a consultant and provide information about what other individuals have done in similar situations, detailing how they became helpers and how, through their activities, they found fulfill-ment.

Some people are able, without the help of a caregiver, to see the challenge hidden in a blow of fate. Joseph Fabry provides this example.

The easy life often seems empty and meaning comes with the chal-lenge to turn defeat into victory. Edward Wilson was a student of English literature at Harvard. He had a brilliant mind that made studying so easy that he was bored. He saw no meaning in life, and in a dark moment shot himself. When he regained consciousness he realized he had failed to kill himself, but that he had blinded himself. While he lay in the hospital, he saw that with this handicap, studying and life would be challenging. Wilson became a teacher and an inspiration for especially gifted students. (Fabry, 1988, p. 89)

Patients with disabling illnesses are uniquely qualified to help others in similar situations. A healthy doctor or family member may be the one to convince a patient in a wheelchair that he or she can still find meaning in life, but another person in a wheelchair or on crutches who is able to say, "I know how you feel because I went through the same trauma myself and found strength I never suspected I had" will be more convincing.

Active Listening is still the caregiver's most valuable tool in helping patients transcend themselves. Asking appropriate open-ended questions that invite the patient to talk, then listening empathically and reflecting back the feelings expressed, invariably will encourage patients to answer their own questions, to find their own meaning in the situation that currently exists.

> Jack, in his mid-sixties, was afflicted with a rare, always fatal, autonomic nervous system disease called Shy-Dragers syndrome. His blood pressure dropped very low when he sat or stood up, and he would rapidly lose consciousness. He was progressively losing control of his limbs, his speech, and his excretory functions. Dorothy, his wife, was caring for him at home with a little help from a home care service. Jack and Dorothy were both overwhelmed with feelings of helplessness and depression. After weeks of intermittent Active Listening (WSE), it became apparent that they wanted desperately to communicate with other people suffering from this same problem. Since they could not find anyone in the local area or the state, they wrote to well-known medical centers where research was being conducted on this disease. In this way they obtained names, addresses, and phone numbers of 25 patients, and soon Dorothy started a telephone support group among caregivers all over the country. This did wonders for her morale, and stimulated Jack's lively interest and participation. They found meaning for themselves and others in sharing feelings in this way.

Those of us who are caregivers must truly believe that patients have their own answers and capabilities within them, and our help should be aimed at *facilitating* their *self-discovery* rather than advising what we think they should do to find meaning in their lives.

Loss of life's meaning may have something to do with the *onset* of certain serious illnesses. In his book *Cancer as a Turning Point*, Lawrence LeShan, a research psychologist, describes the problem as follows:

The single thing that emerged most clearly during my work was the context in which the cancer developed. In a large majority of the patients I saw (certainly not all) there had been, previous to the first noted signs of cancer, a loss of hope in ever achieving a way of life that would give real and deep satisfaction, that would provide a solid raison d'etre, the kind of meaning that makes us glad to get out of bed in the morning and glad to go to bed at night, the kind of life that makes us look forward zestfully to each day and to the future. Often this lack of hope had been brought into being by the loss of the person's major way of relating and expressing himself or herself and the inability to find a meaningful substitute. (1989, p. 106)

It is a well-established statistical fact that widows and widowers develop several types of life-threatening illnesses shortly after the loss of a spouse whom they had made the central focus of their life and the meaning of their existence. The survivors usually could find no other meaning or ways to express themselves. In men, the peak incidence of cancer is shortly after retirement, regardless of age.

Again quoting LeShan:

With many other individuals I saw and worked with there had been no objective loss of relationship, but there had been a loss of hope that the way they used to express themselves and the relationships they had would ever give the deep satisfaction they wanted so much. No matter how successful they were, no matter how high they climbed in their profession, they found that it did not provide fulfillment. They could not find lasting zest and pleasure in their success and eventually had given up hope of ever finding it. The profound hopelessness was in many of the people I saw, followed by the appearance of cancer. (1989, p.106)

LeShan describes a man who retired from a successful business career happy that he could now spend most of his time playing golf and tennis. After a couple of years this life suddenly felt meaningless, and he developed gastric cancer shortly thereafter. He received routine medical treatment and began to work with LeShan to find a new meaning for his life. He finally discovered a new interest in working on world overpopulation problems, which he tackled with enthusiasm. His gastric cancer ceased to be a problem, he felt fulfilled, and he eventually stopped his visits to LeShan because he was too busy.

Everyone can benefit before death by obtaining a clearer understanding of the meaning of one's life. What was it all about? It is not easy to say good-bye to something without knowing what it is. LeShan (1989) describes a way to help people look back over their lives, remembering the good, the bad, the joyful or sad, trying to find the meaning of each of these episodes or relationships from the perspective of someone about to leave. The author (WSE) remembers helping a patient with colon cancer look back and recall what brought him joy and fulfillment:

George, age 66, was still at home, being cared for by his wife who was not well herself. He was yellow as a pumpkin from a liver full of metastatic colon cancer, and his physicians had decided that no further treatment, except pain medication, was likely to be helpful. Over the course of several visits, about two a week, I asked him to tell me about a number of periods of his life—childhood, adolescence, education, his various jobs as an adult. Finally I said to him one day, "George, when you look back over your life as you have done, do you see any meaning, any purpose, any thread running through it?" George thought for a minute and then said, "Look in the back room and tell me what you see." I looked as he instructed, then came back to his living room and said, "I see only a pool table in your back room."

George then said, "When my children were teenagers 20 years ago, the neighborhood kids used to play pool in that room with my kids. My wife and I became almost foster parents to those neighbor children. They discussed their problems, their ambitions with us. Now 20 years later we still get Christmas cards or visits from them when they are in town. You know—I made a difference in those kids' lives, that's what I thought of when you asked about the meaning of my life." George seemed less depressed after that discussion.

Over the last few years the author (WSE) has reviewed their lives and asked this question about meaning of a number of dying individuals, and has gotten various kinds of answers. For a majority, like George, relationships gave meaning more often than financial success or recognition. This facilitative method has proved extremely helpful in encouraging the dying to look back and find purpose and meaning—and sometimes even a feeling of completeness in their remaining time. Sometimes their reminiscences will remind them of relationships that need healing if there is enough time left. This looking back often relaxes the patient; produces calm, lightens depression, and promotes peaceful acceptance of the future. The listener, however, must really be interested and not use this simply as a technique to get the person to talk. Patients are highly sensitive to faked interest and acceptance.

We feel that finding meaning in life can prevent depression and can lead to fulfillment in the remaining days of those with life-threatening illnesses. Caregivers of all kinds can help patients find their own meaning by empathic listening and avoiding Communication Roadblocks.

Chapter 11

Helping the Terminal Patient

Going "gentle into that good night" with one's dignity and sense of self intact is certainly as morally acceptable as raging "against the dying of the light."

— Timothy Quill, 1993, *Death With Dignity*

Roy, a 35-year-old salesman with rapidly progressing leukemia, was being treated as an outpatient, living at home with his wife and two teenage daughters. He was being given excellent emotional support by his family, conversation was open and direct, no one was intimidated by the physical problems, and Roy talked freely about the possibility (even probability) of his dying.

When routine chemotherapy was no longer effective, Roy was hospitalized for more intensive treatment with more powerful drugs. Unfortunately, several complications from these drugs occurred. He developed a bleeding disorder that resulted in a hematoma of the chest wall, a large collection of blood under the skin that had to be opened and drained. This surgical wound became infected and required a long, painful period of daily treatment before it healed. Next, he developed hepatitis, almost certainly from one of the several blood transfusions he was given. This further debilitated him, and he went into a profound depression, became angry at his doctors and his family.

Roy never returned home. He stated that he fervently wished he had not undergone the last series of treatments. He died in the hospital after three months of physical and emotional misery from efforts he had agreed to in hopes that heroic therapy could give him a few more months of life. His experience illustrates the difficulty of deciding whether to keep trying even when there is little hope of a cure, or to accept the inevitability of death and spend the remaining time completing a life with peace and love. A caregiver can be of great help when such decisions must be made by recognizing that it is the patient who owns the problem, and using Active Listening to help the patient find his or her solution to the situation.

If the illness has been prolonged and the patient has worked through denial, anger, and depression, there comes a period when it seems obvious to all that the next stage in the near future is death. This transition may be gradual or rather abrupt, and may or may not be accompanied by increasing pain. There may be a period of acceptance in which the patient relaxes, stops fighting, and lets all concerned know he or she is resigned to letting go. The patient has completed dialogue with family and friends, and may wish to be alone or to have someone sit quietly nearby. This is usually not a happy time; it may be sad but peaceful. Many individuals drift in and out of consciousness as they slide closer to death. In this stage the family and friends may need more support than the patient, and may have more trouble letting go.

This is not a universal description of dying. Some people never quit fighting, never get over their anger at fate or God or themselves. The harder they struggle to avoid the inevitable death, the more they try to deny it, the more difficult it will be for them to reach the final stage of acceptance with peace and dignity. The family and staff may compound the problem by thinking them courageous and encouraging them to fight to the end, and may communicate that giving up is cowardly or a rejection of the family.

Talking about dying is more difficult than it used to be for several reasons. For one thing, our elders seldom die at home, so most people have not experienced death firsthand and it seems unnatural. Even though we intellectually accept the fact that death is inevitable, most of us have not come to accept the certainty of our own death. Another factor is that we have developed such high expectations of medicine that we believe doctors can cure everything. It is shocking to realize this is still a long way from being true. Finally, most of us in developed countries have lost an earlier strong belief in an afterlife that comforted so many of our forebears as death approached.

In spite of recent efforts to humanize the education of young physicians in medical school and residency training, many doctors still are not as good at handling the emotional aspects of dying as they are at caring for the physical aspects of patients' disease. Physicians also are often reluctant to accept the failure of their techniques to save the patient and wish to continue more of the same, although turning the patient to the loving care of friends and family would be much more appropriate. When medical technology has no more to add, friends and family may feel they have already lost their role, and thus remain at a distance, expecting more interventions from the medical team.

Sarah, with advanced breast cancer, was told by her doctor that more chemotherapy would have little chance of helping and that nausea, vomiting, and hair loss would almost certainly result. Her family urged her to keep trying to live, and this pressure was about to win out. An elderly aunt, who was close to the patient, saw what was happening: that the rest of the family wanted Sarah to live for their sakes. By listening at length to Sarah's feelings and reflecting back what she heard, the aunt helped Sarah realize what was happening and then decide against any more treatment. Once the decision was made, the family grew close again and Sarah's last month was relatively painfree. She had long talks with several of the family members with whom she had had conflicts. She had a quiet, peaceful death, and seemed to have reached a feeling of completion.

More suffering is often caused by desperate struggling than by premature acceptance. This is the stage when patients or family reach the "go any-where, try anything" frame of mind. The price paid for this attitude is not only a financial drain but also increased discomfort to the patient and loss of time to be with close friends or family, and the loss of tenderness and sensitivity that might be allowed to grow.

The problem here is that either patient or family, or both, may not yet be ready to give up hope, and may want the medical team to keep trying. The patient's family seems to cling to desperate hope for improvement or cure long after the patient is tired of fighting and has reached the stage of acceptance. This is another appropriate time for Active Listening with family members.

If the alternative suggested is safe, inexpensive, and not too great a drain on the patient's energy stores, it is often helpful for the physician to support its use by using Declarative I-Messages like "I've had no experience with this process, but it might be worth a try." Such therapies as special diets, acupuncture, visualization, and meditation would fall in this category.

To emphasize what was written earlier, patients usually die as they have lived. If they have always been outgoing and friendly, they will continue to live like this to the end; the chronic complainer will continue to be irritable during his or her final days. The major mistake often made by spouses, friends, or professionals is to take over ownership of the problem and try to change the person's attitude so a more peaceful death may occur. This is seldom successful, and it is harmful. This is the language of unacceptance that distances individuals.

To relate to a dying patient, the critical message to get across is one's willingness to listen, first using Declarative I-Messages that disclose you are willing to talk about anything the patient is comfortable with, that you will not be a part of the "conspiracy of silence" unless the patient wants you to be. Also, you can always use an open-ended question such as "How do you feel about what's happening to you?" The patient may complain about the food or nursing care, or may respond with an expression of deeper feelings, depending on his or her level of trust in the speaker, and his or her readiness to acknowledge or accept these deeper feelings. LeShan suggests a number of follow-up, open-ended questions to indicate to the patient that you're comfortable with discussion of feelings at any depth. An exploratory open-ended question may deepen the dialogue: "What is the longest part of the day for you now?" "What occupies your mind at that time?"

The dying person is saying a multitude of good-byes, and friends and family can help by being sensitive to this. Here is another very appropriate time to use Active Listening. The patient is saying good-bye to himself, his aspirations, hopes; good-bye to loved ones, to those he tried to love but could not; even good-bye to goals never to be achieved. Caregivers can encourage discussion of relationships, their incompleteness, what needs to be said to heal these disruptions—these are important avenues toward peace. If possible, finding forgiveness of self as well as of others can be tremendously rewarding, but these feelings are most difficult to achieve without verbalizing them to others who show understanding and acceptance. We listen to our own voices and reach new emotional insights more by *talking* through the problem than by *thinking* through the problem alone.

As George, who was dying of advanced colon cancer, approached the terminal stage, he was admitted to the hospice unit at the VA medical center, where the author (WSE) visited him frequently. He began to sleep most of the time but was quite lucid while awake. The following conversation was stimulated by an open-ended question.

WSE: George, I've never been where you are, what is it like?

G (with a faint smile): I don't see any tunnel with a bright light at the end. I feel tired but peaceful. I've said everything I want to say to my wife and sons, and I'm ready to go. Unfortunately, they keep encouraging me to keep trying to stay alive, and I wish they would relax.

WSE: Do you mind if I tell them that?

G: No, I wish you would.

I spoke to the family, who had waited in the visitors' lounge while I visited George. They were a little surprised by George's request, but agreed to talk with him and accept his wishes. George died that night.

Ethics committees can often be helpful in decision making, as in the case of John.

John was an 85-year-old widower with advanced prostate cancer causing progressive kidney failure and severe bone pain. The family raised the question of instituting dialysis. They (two sons and a daughter) wanted it. The patient couldn't decide but was not anxious to have the surgery required to allow the connections to the dialysis equipment. The doctors advised against it because it would only prolong a very painful existence for a few days or weeks at most, and would offer no chance for cure or improvement in his basic problem, the prostate cancer.

This situation, which is common these days, produces legal, ethical, and relationship problems that are difficult to resolve. Legally, patients themselves, if mentally competent, should make the decision. How do you judge mental competence? If the patient can tell you his name, age, address, the current date, and the name of the current president of the United States, does that mean he or she is competent to make therapy decisions? Must a physician yield to the pressure of a patient or family to try heroic measures the physician knows will not be useful? Once started, must these heroic measures be continued indefinitely, even if the patient is comatose or not showing improvement? Most hospitals now have ethics committees that do not make decisions but can help with communication between all parties, hoping to produce no-lose decisions that will satisfy everyone.

In John's case, the ethics committee arranged a meeting with the patient, his family, and his physicians. Each person presented his or her needs, opinions, and recommendations, after which a consensus developed that dialysis and other more aggressive measures were no longer indicated, and that vigorous pain management and comfort care were the highest priorities. John and his family became convinced that this was the direction his case should take. John went home with one of his sons and received hospice support until his death three weeks later.

Patient autonomy is now being honored by the medical profession and by courts. Physicians and hospitals are encouraging all persons, especially those who are elderly or chronically ill, to prepare advance directives or living wills indicating whether they want to be treated with heroic measures in the event of terminal illness when the patient is not mentally competent to make such a decision. Advance directives, if available, may be of significant help to the medical team and the family when the patient is near death, but they often are not broad enough to cover all situations. For instance, if a comatose, elderly patient develops pneumonia, would the patient have wanted to prolong this state with antibiotic treatment? Usually this kind of problem is not included under "heroic treatment," so the physicians and family are not helped by the living will. A more useful arrangement may be for the patient, while still competent, to select a family member or trusted friend to be given a durable health power of attorney. This individual should become knowledgeable about as many situations as possible and try to understand the patient's choices in each. Many states have passed laws making living wills and the health power of attorney legal and enforceable.

Many health professionals are reluctant to talk about their own dying or to bring up the prospect of others facing death, so there are still very many patients who reach a terminal stage with mental confusion and no one knowing what choices they would make. This leads to family conflicts and conflicts between family and the medical team.

If you are the caregiver and want to discuss the patient's wishes, the best way to encourage discussion on the part of the patient is to use self-disclosure—bring up your own feelings on the subject, then encourage the patient to share his or her opinion, as in this example:

My parents left us no instructions about their wishes before they became mentally confused, so we didn't know what they would have wanted over their last several years. To prevent this, I've written out my wishes for my family, indicating that I don't want any treatment to prolong life if I become irreversibly mentally incompetent. I just want comfort care and pain management, no antibiotics, no intravenous feeding, etc. I wonder how you feel about this problem. Have you thought about such decisions? I'd like to know your wishes.

Again, the use of self-disclosure to express your own feelings, followed by Active Listening, will help patients get in touch with their own deeper feelings more than any other technique available.

For many years, a major goal of medicine, and of doctors and nurses, has been to keep the patient alive as long as possible, regardless of the pain, indignity, and discomfort the patient might suffer. Death of a patient was looked on as a failure, regardless of how welcome it was to the patient or family. Technology has now allowed physicians to keep people alive well past the point of compassion and sensitivity. Physicians are struggling with the legalities and ethical considerations of when to let go. Advance directives can be very helpful, as indicated earlier, but more and more often these days another dilemma arises—the patient begins to consider ending life by suicide because he or she perceives only a long, painful road ahead. In many such situations the patient may ask the doctor to assist in this final act by writing a prescription or giving an injection. Doctors are prevented by law and by ethics from assisting suicide in an overt way, but it is permissible to discontinue machines and drugs that can no longer hope to cure. At this period in history many people with AIDS are considering or practicing suicide to eliminate the long, slow process of dying. Physicians must determine their level of comfort in dealing with this issue. It is clear that many people, especially the elderly, are anxious to have some control over their dying, not leaving it entirely up to the medical team.

Derek Humphrey's book *Final Exit* (1991), a surprise best-seller, gave people a method of escape and a feeling of control. Quite probably there would be less use or need of suicide if last days could be made more painfree and comfortable, and especially less lonely. Two recent developments have made this more practical. The first is the hospice movement, which provides comfort care only for the dying—in a special unit of a hospital or at home, whichever patients choose. To be a candidate for hospice care, a medical guess must be made that the patient has a life expectancy of six months or less.

The second movement, even more recent, is the beginnings of a new medical specialty of palliative care for those for whom cure is no longer possible. Only a few such fellowship training programs are now available, but several more are in the planning stage.

The U.S. medical system has been slow to accept palliative care and the hospice concept. Referrals from attending physicians or even from private oncologists are few—most are from neighbors, family members, or friends. Physicians, as well as patients and families, hate to give up hope.

Another deficiency in the medical system and its treatment of those who can't be cured is that many physicians don't treat pain very well. In the words of a physician, "I'm afraid of producing addiction or having the patient need bigger and bigger doses, or even taking an overdose. It's better in my opinion to let the patient have a little pain than to risk these complications." This has been the prevailing philosophy of physicians for many years. Addiction, tolerance, and intentional overdoses are not serious problems in the dying. Pain management is under study, and researchers are learning more about how to relieve pain without making the patient drowsy or confused. Using the participation principle, more and more physicians are giving patients control of their pain medications within what are considered safe limits. Family caregivers should be aware of this and request patient control if this is possible.

Dying patients usually know before the family does that the end is near, and they are ready to let go. This can be quite sad if it prevents saying loving good-byes. It seems more mistakes are made by trying desperately to keep someone alive than by letting go too soon. This, too, is gradually changing.

We would like to conclude this chapter with two wonderful quotes. Five days before he died in 1981, William Saroyan called the Associated Press to leave this statement: "Everybody has got to die but I have always believed an exception would be made in my case. Now what?" And Ronald Reagan's remark as he was wheeled into surgery with a gunshot wound of the chest: "I hope the surgeon is a Republican." Such humor shows how alive one can be even in the face of death.

Chapter 12

Other Applications of Interpersonal Skills

All of the communication skills and the problem-solving and conflict resolution procedures we have described and illustrated in previous chapters are equally effective in other relationships and in other settings. Their effectiveness has been repeatedly proven in families, in classrooms, in the workplace. In this final chapter the authors will point out some other applications that may be of special interest to health professionals.

HEALTH PROFESSIONALS AS GROUP LEADERS

Obviously, physicians not only relate to their patients but also must interact with the members of their office staff. In fact, many medical offices are not unlike a work group in a business organization, with a leader and group members. Some may consist of two or more physicians in a partnership plus their employees. No matter how a medical office looks on an organization chart, it involves people relating to each other. Referring back to our Behavior Window, employees will inevitably experience problems they own that call for Active Listening by physicians, and their behaviors can cause problems for physicians that call for nonblameful, Confrontive I-Messages or No-Lose Conflict Resolution.

Physicians in medical offices must do a lot of teaching—giving instructions, explaining new procedures, and doing on-the-job training of staff members. Teaching others may seem like a simple and straightforward task of correcting employees' performance and showing them a better way, but it's seldom that easy. Group members often respond to their leaders' teaching with resistance, defensiveness, embarrassment, irritation, and sometimes anger:

I hope I don't forget.

What's wrong with my way?

Dr. Jenkins wanted it done like this.

Nobody told me anything different.

I could never learn that way; I must be dumb.

It goes without saying that such responsive messages call for the teacher to show empathic understanding and acceptance by using Active Listening.

Sometimes health professionals as leaders will have an opportunity to contribute to the personal growth of a group member by using Active Listening to help the person work through a problem and wind up with new insights or effective solutions. A brief counseling session with employees can bring about significant and lasting improvements of their performance: a shy employee is helped to speak up more frequently in office meetings; a nurse gets insight into the causes of her carelessness and takes remedial action; a compulsive and perfectionistic bookkeeper relaxes her unrealistic standards, as in the following dialogue with her boss, Hal. Initially she was troubled by her heavy workload, but Active Listening helped her discover the more basic problem:

Cathy: I hate the feeling of being behind and not pulling my weight. It makes me feel guilty when I go home at night.

Hal: So it's really getting to you.

Cathy: I'm conscientious. I like to do good and accurate work. Sometimes I think I'm too conscientious—too much a stickler for accuracy.

Hal: Sounds like you're proud of your work and want to make it absolutely top-notch, but you're beginning to wonder if you're putting in too much time and effort on making it superterrific.

Cathy: Yeah, I think so. There are times when I go over my figures three or four times, when down deep inside I know that's unnecessary, because I seldom find a mistake. But there's something in me that says, "Well, I'd better do it again, because I don't want anybody catching me making a mistake."

Hal: Well, it sounds like you're really realizing that you overdo your checking, but something inside of you . . . some fear of getting caught in a mistake . . . just compels you to keep on checking.

Cathy: Yeah, I've always been that way. Not just about my work; I'm that way about lots of things. I guess you might say I'm kind of a perfectionist.

Hal: So you're seeing this as a theme throughout your whole life. That you just have to be free of blame and perfect all the time.

Cathy: Yeah, but it's often a real burden because it takes time to be perfect. And it's as if sometimes I'm cutting my nose off to spite my face. I miss out on doing a lot of things, because I feel I shouldn't do them unless I do them perfectly.

Hal: So this desire to be perfect is really preventing you from doing more things and having a richer life.

Cathy: Yeah, I'm beginning to see that's true. For a long time, I've really wanted to play tennis, and two months ago I signed up for lessons.

Hal: No kidding.

Cathy: And my friends call me up to ask me to play, and I really like to play, but I say, "No, I don't want to play." The reason I say that is because I want to get more lessons so that I'll have more confidence.

Hal: I understand.

Cathy: So that when I do play with my friends, they don't see that I make mistakes, or I guess I want them to see how good I am.

Hal: Uh . . . it almost sounds like you're seeing this . . . this need to look good is preventing you from making social contacts and having fun, and being free, and it's cutting out a lot of fun in life.

Cathy: That's right. Going back to my work, if I could get less compulsive about having to have everything perfect, I'm sure I'd get more done.

Hal: You almost sound like you have an idea for a solution to part of your problem, and that is to cut down on some of your worrying and checking. You're going to see how it goes.

Cathy: Yeah, because there're some things that just aren't worth three or four checks. There might be one mistake, that really isn't catastrophic, I think, in our business. (Pause)

Hal: I get it.

Cathy: In bookkeeping, there are so many cross-checks that it isn't necessary for me to go over every column of figures . . . over and over again.

Hal: I see.

Cathy: I just think it has slowed me down.

Hal: So you can see there really wouldn't be as much of a penalty involved, if you let a mistake slip by every six months, as you've been imagining.

Cathy: Right.

Hal: That sounds like you're kind of working up your courage to test out that hypothesis.

Cathy: I'd like to give it a try for a week and see whether I can make this change. I'm not sure I can, but it makes so much sense to me, I'd like to give it a try, and get back to you if some other solution needs to be worked out. I think I'll go back and give it a try. Thanks for listening.

Hal: You're sure welcome. I feel real good about this conversation.

Health professionals, in their role as leaders of their office staffs, should seriously consider adopting the same collaborative model in relationships with their staff members as we prescribed for their relationships with patients. To build this kind of relationship with group members, health professionals need all the skills we have described in previous chapters. These skills will help establish a climate of acceptance in the group that will foster more member participation in problem-solving staff meetings.

The leader's goal might be described as becoming more like a group member while helping group members become more like a group leader. However, finding the appropriate balance between encouraging the full participation of group members and contributing one's own ideas in group meetings can be a problem for many leaders. But that is also a problem for each group member. In fact, both must find a balance between listening to others and self-disclosure.

Health professionals who are successful in developing collaborative relationships and building their employees into an effective problem-solving team will certainly *prevent* many of the typical conflicts that occur in groups with authoritarian leadership. Nevertheless, some conflicts will happen even in the most democratic of groups. As a group leader a health professional can count on becoming involved with a wide variety of conflicts—with an individual group member, with several members, or with the total staff team. In such situations, the six-step No-Lose Conflict Resolution Method will be invaluable. Not only will conflicts be resolved amicably, but the process itself creates a group climate in which all members feel it is safer to identify and expose conflicts rather than suppress them.

If health professionals apply interpersonal skills as leaders of their medical office staff, they will find that they are truly making staff members their partners. As a result, relationships within the group will deepen and become more satisfying. Communication between members will become more open, honest, and direct. Problems will be brought to the surface, where they will be recognized and resolved.

Over time, sometimes in a surprisingly short time, leadership in the group will become distributed—moving away from the formal leader, the physician, and toward the group members. Instead of top management having to set goals for staff members, and then use rewards and punishments to control the members' behavior and monitor their progress toward those goals, physicians will be able to create work groups in which the spotlight and the locus of control are shifted away from a patriarchal boss and toward the group members. The alternative authoritarian leadership, inevitably fosters dependency or rebellion, which make partnerships unattainable.

However, it is the strong conviction of both authors of this book that a high level of effectiveness as a group-centered or democratic leader is not as likely to be achieved by a health professional without participating in a well-designed training program that has a proven record of success in teaching the critical skills and procedures necessary to build collaborative relationships.

For almost four decades one of the authors (TG) has been involved in such activity. Initially doing this training himself, then later training and authorizing other instructors, his *Leader Effectiveness Training* course has been taught in countries to several hundred thousand leaders—school administrators, managers and supervisors in business and government organizations, ministers, physicians, and dentists. (See Appendix, page 199.)

FAMILY MEMBERS AS CAREGIVERS

The interpersonal skills we have described and illustrated throughout this book are equally applicable and valuable to persons who assume the role of a caregiver for a family member with a chronic illness or a life-threatening disease. Whether they are parents, children, spouses, or other relatives, such patients inevitably experience a wide range of feelings—confusion, fear, pain, loneliness, depression, hopelessness, anxiety, anger. They may also suffer a loss of sexual prowess, independence, confidence, and self-esteem.

Serious illness can weaken the strength of a marriage, and it can have serious effects on the family members who are forced to take on new roles and obligations. In fact, a person with a serious illness may be the most critical factor in the psychological health of the other family members. Nothing could be more valuable and effective to help family members meet this test than knowing the interpersonal communication skills, the problem-ownership concept, the participation principle, the six-step problem-solving process and the conflict-resolution methodology.

Proof of the effectiveness of these skills and procedures has come from a number of parents who, after taking the Parent Effectiveness Training (P.E.T.) course, have used the skills they learned to help youngsters with serious illnesses. The following story was submitted to the author (TG) by a mother whose child had cystic fibrosis. Here is her story in her own words:

Cystic fibrosis is a serious lung disease. Often it is fatal before the age of 18. Mark had been diagnosed at three, a week before his infant sister died of the same disease. Children with CF produce a thick, sticky mucus that clogs the ducts of the pancreas and other body organs. In the pancreas it creates difficult digestive problems. Most devastating is what that mucus does in the lungs and bronchial tree—blocking tiny areas, setting up infections that can mean gradual deterioration of the lungs. It's a constant battle with antibiotics and therapy to keep those lung infections in check.

With Mark, as with many others who have CF, it is often a losing battle. Each year he's spent more and more time in the hospital. His daily bucket of pills ranges between 40 and 50. He is unable to go without antibiotics.

Mark knows he has trouble running. Two years ago he gave up playing Little League. He knows kids die of CF, because some of the friends he met at the hospital have died. Obviously he knows he can't do as much this year as he did a year or two back. We've kind of accepted that, without talking about it much. Actually, I think we spent years talking around it.

I'd been wanting Mark to have his say on the subject of CF, but I didn't think he wanted to talk about it—he'd never brought the subject up—or more likely, I'd never heard the clues. That night I did.

He said he wanted to thank me for the poem I'd written him and the card I'd made for him. I explained how I'd looked everywhere for just the right gift, but kept remembering how he'd always said he disliked it when people bought gifts just because it was a special day. I told him I'd been afraid to share the poem with him because it was happy/sad writing. He nodded. "But," I said, "I decided to trust you with my thoughts because it kept coming to my mind that it was the gift that would mean the most." Not just to him, but to me also.

He started talking then about the importance of people sharing what is real with each other, and how many people he sees that are phonies. His voice went from disgust to anger. He spoke in bitter words against the people in school and in our church, making accusations I felt were too harsh about "those damned Sunday Christians." It became very hard for me to listen. I had to fight my impulse to defend those people, to ask him to be more kind toward them.

When I didn't stop him, he said more. Now it was not just the people, it was also the teachings of the church that were "stupid." Then it was that people were cruel. "Where do they get all their answers on how to live a beautiful long life" he spit out angrily.

I was getting really uptight. I couldn't remember having heard him swear before. He did now. "They think they're so goddamned smart," and "How in the hell do they know what it's like to be different?"

I was afraid I couldn't stand to hear any more. My throat felt like it had needles in it, and when I realized how tightly my hand was clutching the kitchen chair, I also knew how badly my feet wanted to carry me away to another place. I kept saying to my head: "Don't buy into the problem. Let him own his own feelings so you can listen to them."

Finally he just broke down and sobbed. He pounded the table so hard I was afraid he'd hurt himself, and he screamed, "I'm afraid to die. I don't want to die."

After moments that seemed like hours, as I wondered what to do now, he lifted his head from his arms and met my eyes.

"I had to say that, Mom," he said. We hugged each other and cried together. Then, after we'd sat in silence for a while, he looked up, half sheepishly and said, "Well, let's get those dishes done now."

Just like that.

If I'd been directing the scene, as parents are so wont to do, I'd have probably suggested I'd come up to his room and say good night. Mark was having none of that. It was midnight as we washed those dishes and talked about our feelings and fears. Many of them, we discovered, were honestly very joyful. It felt like a celebration. Like we were having communion together over the kitchen sink. And why not?

"I feel so good," Mark kept saying. He told me he was happy I'd be teaching P.E.T. "That stuff is really important," he said. "You know, sometime maybe I could help you out with it."

He already had. Maybe more than he'll ever know. (Gordon, 1976, pp. 289–92)

A father submitted the following report of his experience of finding Active Listening of great value in dealing with his adolescent son, who at age 14 discovered he had diabetes.

I took P.E.T. from Dr. Gordon in 1965 because my 15-year-old son, the oldest, was having a great deal of trouble during his adolescence. And, after the second or third session of the course, my wife and I became very enthusiastic about what we were learning. Then between the fourth and fifth session a dramatic occurrence happened to us.

Our youngest son, Brian, who was only 14 at the time, was diagnosed with a severe case of diabetes. In fact, we got him to the hospital just in time to keep him from going into a diabetic coma. After my wife and Brian and I had weathered the shock of this illness and it came time to bring Brian home from the hospital, the doctor told us that Brian would have to give himself a shot before he left the hospital. They had him practicing giving oranges hypodermic shots, but he seemed unable to give himself one.

The doctor also told us that we were in for two or three years of very difficult sledding with this young boy because the typical course of diabetes is that the young person who has contracted the disease becomes emotionally unstable, with lots of depression and defiance. He predicted that he would probably go off his strict diet and refuse to give himself shots, and would probably wind up in the hospital in a diabetic coma at least two or three times before the next several years had passed.

Well, this seemed like a terrible problem to us. So one evening we sat down and looked at the P.E.T. course and what we had learned. We reviewed the concept of "who owns the problem," and since it was definitely Brian's body that was having the problem, he obviously owned the problem. Then we recalled that the skill recommended by P.E.T. when the other person owned the problem was Active Listening. Before this, we had been emotionally set to coerce him to give himself a shot, give him all kinds of advice about the need for him to stay on his case, and monitor him closely to be sure he got well.

When we accepted the reality of his owning the problem and recalled that Active Listening is the preferred skill to use, we said to each other that if Active Listening was going to work, it was going to work here—an acid test of Active Listening as far as we were concerned. We decided that we were going to use this skill anytime he had problems or difficulties. First, we decided to bring him home from the hospital after listening to him say that he was too afraid to give himself a shot. Fortunately, we were able to talk the hospital into releasing him into our custody. Brian immediately found a diabetic friend who told him that he had found a little mechanical gadget that was spring-loaded. When you put the syringe in and held it against your skin and pulled the trigger, the machine shot the needle into you. You didn't have to do it yourself. So he immediately had us go out and buy him one of these. That day he gave himself his first shot using this mechanical device. After that, he took full charge of his diet even though he had some depression about it. Understandably it must be depressing to find out you have a disease that is going to last all of your life, that you're going to be giving yourself insulin shots all the rest of your life, and that the disease will have some devastating side effects as you grow older. We knew it was a daunting prospect for a young adolescent to face.

So we continued to do a lot of Active Listening. As a result, he got over a lot of his depression. He even managed his diet by himself. We never had to remind him of that. But after a few weeks, he got really depressed one day. I was sitting in his room, and as I was listening to him, I recognized that he was more depressed than usual. I did my best as an Active Listener, but it got pretty frightening for me when he got to the point where it sounded to me like he was considering suicide. In fact, he said, "Dad, I am so devastated by having this terrible disease that I really, really feel like ending it all." Hearing this, I was really frightened and was tempted to use all the Roadblocks in the book: "Brian, don't even think of it," "Brian, it'll look better to you tomorrow." "This is just a phase you're going through." And so forth. But I gritted my teeth and thought, "Ralph, if you're ever going to Active Listen, do it now." So I fed back his feelings as best I could: "Brian, you hate your body so much that you'd like to kill it." I sat there, and I started to sweat and look at the floor. And after a while he said, "Yeah." Then I sat there, shaking inside, and waited some more. Finally he looked up and said, "But I don't think I have the nerve to do that, Dad, so I guess I better just get on with it." He got up and went over to a friend's house, and that was the last we ever heard of his idea to kill himself.

These two dramatic examples of parents using their communication skills in the role of caregivers for their children with serious health problems illustrate how effective parents can be after being trained in communication skills. Physicians could suggest to caregivers that *they* might learn the interpersonal skills—from this book or other books that teach these skills. (See Appendix, page 199.)

Health professionals should also be aware of the existence of successful peer counseling programs in their community, particularly those serving the needs of older people with mental or physical health problems. One such program known to the author (TG) was created in Santa Monica, California, by Evelyn Freeman in 1976. Called the Senior Health and Peer Counseling Center (SHPCC), its model is being replicated throughout the United States, Canada, and Denmark. Agencies that have adopted the SHPCC training model have trained counselors to deal with a broad range of problems:

Mental health problems

Physical and medical problems, including strokes, Alzheimer's disease and other forms of dementia

Multiple sclerosis

Vision and hearing impairments

Concerns of frail, isolated, institutionalized, and homebound patients

Substance abuse

Problems of ethnic minorities

Concerns related to gender.

The training offered in the SHPCC model stresses empathic listening, group leadership skills, and just being with the person rather than doing something for him or her. (See Appendix, page 199.)

Undoubtedly it is already clear to the reader that all the skills and procedures the authors have described and illustrated throughout the book are applicable in all person-to-person relationships—in families, in schools, in the workplace. In fact, a considerable amount of research evidence strongly shows that our system of skills and procedures we have recommended for health professionals is in fact a generic system that fosters health, well-being, happiness, and mutual need satisfaction in all relationships.

Parents who learn the system to improve their relationship with their children invariably report they use all the skills and methods in their marriage relationship. Managers and supervisors who have been trained to use the system to develop effective work teams and good relationships with their subordinates frequently report that they are applying the system at home with their children. Salespeople find the system invaluable in creating long-term win-win partnerships with their customers (Zaiss and Gordon, 1993). The system is also being used in training programs for schoolteachers, probation officers, youth workers, ministers, and other professionals.

We are aware of the growing interest within the medical and nursing professions in training for the improvement of relationships with patients. We hope our book will reinforce and accelerate this important movement within the various health care professions.

Sources of Information about Communication Skills Training for Health Professionals

MEDICAL GROUPS

American Academy on Physician and Patient
Mack Lipkin, Jr., M.D., President
New York University Medical Center
Department of Medicine
550 First Avenue
New York, NY 10016
1-212-263-8291

The Society of Teachers of Family Medicine
Group on Doctor–Patient Interaction
P.O. Box 8729
Kansas City, MO 64114
1-800-274-2237

The Health Communication Research Institute, Inc.
Marlene M. von Friedrichs-Fitzwater, Ph.D., Director
1050 Fulton Ave., Suite #105
Sacramento, CA 95825
1-916-974-8686

"Caring through Communication" Workshops
Ann C. Jobe, M.D., Coordinator, Patient Physician Project
East Carolina State University School of Medicine
Brody Medical Science Building
Greeneville, NC 27858–4354
1-919-816-2278

Miles Institute for Health Care Communications, Inc.
J. Gregory Carroll, Ph.D., Director
400 Morgan Lane
West Haven, CT 06516
1-800-800-5907

RECOMMENDED BOOKS

Annotated bibliography of doctor-patient communication of the Task Force on Doctor and Patient (1992) (now the American Academy on Physician and Patient) Second Edition, by Scott Sherman, Samuel Putnam, Mack Lipkin, Aaron Lazare, John Stoeckle, Vaughn Keller, and J. Gregory Carroll. New York: Miles Institute for Health Care Communications, Inc. An annotated bibliography of 125 of the best works in this area, recently updated by the American Academy on Physician and Patient.

Be your best: Personal effectiveness in your life and your relationships (1989), by Linda Adams. New York: Putnam. A thorough presentation of the interpersonal skills and conflict-resolution procedures essential for creating any mutually satisfying relationship.

Communicating with medical patients (1989), edited by Moira Stewart and Debra Roter. Newbury Park: Sage Publications. Results of a ground-breaking conference in which diverse scholars of the interview work together to find common ground.

Doctors talking with patients/Patients talking with doctors (1992), by Debra L. Roter and Judith A. Hall. Westport, CT: Auburn House. Based upon an extensive body of research (248 references), this book provides an in-depth analysis of the doctor-patient relationship, the patterns of talk in the medical visit, the prospects for improving communication, and the relationship of talk to patient outcomes.

Leader effectiveness training (1977), by Thomas Gordon, Ph.D. New York: G. P. Putnam's Sons. This book provides a comprehensive system of leadership skills and procedures necessary for health professionals who want to get their employees or members of their medical team to work more effectively and collaboratively, resolve their conflicts amicably, and make their meetings more productive. It is the textbook for Dr. Gordon's L.E.T. workshops, widely used by hundreds of major corporations.

The medical interview: Clinical care, education, research (1995), edited by Mack Lipkin, Samuel Putnam, and Aaron Lazare. New York: Springer-Verlag. A 50-chapter, empirically-based, definitive discussion of the medical interview. With over 70 authors and 1,300 references, this book provides specific detailed approaches to the major doctor-patient interactional situations. The major sections are: A Framework for the Medical Interview; The Structure and Process of the Medical Interview; The Context of the Interview; Specific Interview Situations; Values, Ethics, and Legal Issues; Teaching and Faculty Development; Evaluation of the Interview; and Research on the Medical Interview.

For information about Dr. Gordon's workshops that offer interpersonal training to doctors, nurses and other health professionals, write or phone:

Thomas Gordon, Ph.D.
Effectiveness Training International
531 Stevens Avenue
Solana Beach, CA 92075
1-800-628-1197

Bibliography

Adams, L. (1989). *Be your best*. New York: Putnam.

Allen, L., and Gorski, R. (1992). Sexual orientation and the size of the anterior commissure in the human brain. *Proc. Natl. Acad. Sci. USA*, *89*, 7199–7202.

Allport, G. (1945). The psychology of participation. *Psychol. Rev.*, *53*, 117–132.

Ballard-Reisch, D. (1990). A model of participative decision-making for physician–patient interaction. *Health Communication, 2*.

Barbour, A. (1975). Humanistic patient care: A comparison of the disease model and the growth model. In S. Miller et al., *Dimensions of humanistic medicine*. San Francisco: Institute: Institute for the Study of Humanistic Medicine.

Bauman, K., and Hale, F. (1985). Bringing the homosexual out: Teaching the doctor role. *Med. Educ.*, *11*, 459–462.

Baumrind, D. (1967). Child care practices anteceding three patterns of pre-school behavior. *Genetic Psych. Monog.*, *75*, 43–88.

Beckman, H., and Frankel, R. (1984). The effect of physician behavior on the collection of data. *Ann. Int. Med.*, *101*, 692–696.

Belknap, M.; Blau, R.; and Grossman, R. (1975). *Case studies and methods in humanistic medical care*. San Francisco: Institute for the Study of Humanistic Medicine, 27–28.

Bellet, P., and Maloney, M. (1991). The importance of empathy as an interviewing skill in medicine. *JAMA*, *266*, 1831–1832.

Bertakis, K. (1977). The communication of information from physician to patient: A method for increasing patient retention and satisfaction. *J. Fam. Pract.*, *5*, 217–222.

Bird, J., and Cohen-Cole, S. (1990). The three function model of the medical interview. In M. Hale, ed., Methods in teaching consultation-liason psychiatry. *Adv. Psychosom. Med.*, *20*, 65–88.

Bloom, J., and Spiegel, D. (1989). The relationships of two dimensions of social support to the psychological well being and social functioning of women with advanced breast cancer. *Soc. Sci. Med.*, *19*, 831–837.

Bolton, R. (1979). *People skills.* New York: Simon and Schuster.

Brody, D. (1980). The patient's role in clinical decision-making. *Ann. Int. Med.*, *93*, 718–722.

Brown, K. (1990). The nurse, empathy, and patient satisfaction. Ph.D. diss., University of Utah.

Buckman, R. (1988). *I don't know what to say.* Boston: Little Brown.

Cassell, E. (1985). *Talking with patients.* Vol. 1, *The theory of doctor–patient communication.* Cambridge: MIT Press.

Chelune, G. (1979). *Self-disclosurer.* San Francisco: Jossey-Bass.

Comstock, L.; Hooper, E.; Goodwin, J. M.; and Goodwin, J. S. (1982). Physician behaviors that correlate with patient satisfaction. *J. Med. Educ.*, *57*, 105–112.

Cook, M. (1990). Physician risk and responsibility in the HIV epidemic. *West. J. Med.*, *152*, 57–61.

Cousins, Norman. (1979). *Anatomy of an illness.* New York: W. W. Norton.

———. (1989). *Head first: The biology of hope.* New York: E. P. Dutton.

Crouch, M., and McCauley, J. (1986). Interviewing style and response to family information by family practice residents. *Fam. Med.*, *18*, 15–18.

Daigneault, R. (1993). Personal correspondence with author.

Delbanco, T. (1993). The healing roles of doctor and patient. In B. Moyers, *Healing and the mind.* New York: Doubleday.

Deutsch, M. (1985). *Distributive justice: A social-psychological perspective.* New Haven: Yale University Press.

DiMatteo, M. (1985). Physician–patient communication promoting a positive health-care setting. In J. Rosen and L. Solomon, eds., *Prevention in health psychology.* Hanover, N.H.: University Press of New England.

———. (1991). *The psychology of health, illness, and medical care.* Pacific Grove, Calif.: Brooks/Cole.

Emanuel, E., and Emanuel, L. (1992). Four models of the physician–patient relationship. *JAMA*, *267*, 2221–2226.

Fabry, J. (1988). *Guideposts to meaning.* Oakland, Calif.: New Harbing Publications.

Fisher, S. (1986). *In the patient's best interest: Women and the politics of medical decisions.* New Brunswick: Rutgers University Press.

Frankl, V. (1959). *Man's search for meaning.* New York: Pocket Books/Simon and Schuster.

Gerberding, J.; Bryant-LeBlanc, C.; et al. (1987). Risk of transmitting the HIV, CmV and hepatitis B virus to health care workers exposed to patients with AIDS and AIDS related conditions. *J. Infect. Dis.*, *156*, 1–8.

Gerberding, J.; Littell, B.; Tarkington, A.; Brown, A.; and Schecter, W. (1990). Risk of exposure of surgical personnel to patients' blood during surgery at San Francisco General Hospital. *NEJM*, *332*, 1788–1793.

Gerrard, B.; Boniface, W.; and Love, B. (1980). *Interpersonal skills for health professionals*. Reston, Va.: Reston Publishing Co.

Goldman, J. (1987). An elective seminar to teach first-year medical students the social and medical aspects of AIDS. *J. Med. Educ.*, *62*, 557–561.

Gordon, T. (1955). *Group-centered leadership*. Boston: Houghton Mifflin.

————. (1970). *Parent effectiveness training*. New York: Penguin Books.

————. (1974). *Teacher effectiveness training*. New York: David McKay.

————. (1976). *P.E.T. in action*. New York: Perigree Books.

————. (1977). *Leader effectiveness training*. New York: Putnam.

Granoff, M. (1970). An analysis of meanings and consequences of self-disclosing behavior. Ph.D. diss., University of Texas.

Guerney, B. (1982). *Relationship enhancement*. San Francisco: Jossey-Bass.

Guerney, B.; Brock, G.; and Coutal, J. (1986). Integrating marital therapy and enrichment: The relationship enhancement approach. In N. Jacobson and S. Gurman, eds., *Clinical handbook of marital therapy*. Guilford Press.

Hall, J.; Roter, D.; and Katz, N. (1988). Meta-analysis of correlates of provider behavior in medical encounters. *Med. Care*, *26*, 657–675.

Helfer, R. (1970). An objective comparison of the pediatric interviewing skills of freshman and senior medical students. *Pediatrics*, *45*, 623–627.

Henbest, R., and Fehrsen, G. (1992). Patient-centeredness: Is it applicable outside the west? Its measurement and effect on outcomes. *Fam. Prac.*, *9*, 311–317.

Humphrey, D. (1991). *Final exit*. Eugene, Oreg.: Humane Society.

Jay, J., and Young, A. (1979). *The gay reports*. New York: Summit Books.

Johnson, D.; Marvyama, G.; Johnson, R.; Nelson, D.; and Skon, L. (1981). Effects of cooperative, competitive and individualistic goal structures on achievement: A meta-analysis. *Psychol. Bull.*, *89*, 47–62.

Jourard, S. (1964). *The transparent self*. New York: D. Van Nostrand.

Jourard, S. (1971). *The transparent self*. (Revised edition). New York: D. Van Nostrand.

Kastenbaum, R., and Aisenberg, R. (1972). *The psychology of death*. New York: Springer.

Kelly, J.; St. Lawrence, J.; Smith, S.; et al. (1987). Medical students' attitude toward AIDS and homosexual patients. *J. Med. Educ.*, *62*, 549–556.

Koop, C. E. (1992). *Monitor*, American Psychological Association. Oct., p. 5.

Korsch, B., and Negrete, V. (1972). Doctor–patient communication. *Sci. Amer.*, *227*, 66–74.

Krupan, E. (1986). A delicate balance. *Psych. Today*, Nov., pp. 22–26.

Kübler-Ross, E. (1969). *On death and dying*. New York: Macmillan.

Kus, R. (1988). Alcoholism and non-acceptance of gay self: The critical link. *J. Homosexuality, 15*, 23–41.

———. (1990). *Keys to caring: Assisting your gay and lesbian clients*. Boston: Alyson.

LeShan, L. (1989). *Cancer as a turning point*. New York: E. P. Dutton.

Lester, G., and Smith, S. (1993). Listening and talking to patients—a remedy for malpractice suits? *West. J. Med., 158*, 268–272.

LeVay, S. (1991). A difference in hypothalamic structure between heterosexual and homosexual men. *Science, 253*, 1034–1037.

Levenstein, J.; Brown, J.; Weston, W.; Stewart, M.; McCracken, E.; and McWhinney, I. (1989). Patient-centered clinical interviewing. In M. Stewart and D. Roger, eds. *Communication with medical patients*. Beverly Hills: Sage.

Levy, D. (1985). White doctors and black patients: Influence of race on the doctor–patient relationship. *Pediatrics, 75*, 4, 639–643.

Ley, P. (1988). *Communication with patients*. New York: Croom Helm.

Lipkin, M.; Quill, T.; and Napadano, R. (1984). The medical interview: A core curriculum for residencies in internal medicine. *Ann. Int. Med., 100*, 2, 277–284.

Lown, B.; DeSilva, R.; Reich, P.; and Murawski, B. (1980). Psychophysiological factors in sudden cardiac death. *Am. J. Psych., 137*, 1325–1335.

Manuel, P. (1993). Personal communication to author.

McCollum, S. (1992). Healing: A broader definition of success. Speech to medical students, University Hospital Learning Center, Albuquerque, N. Mex.

McCrory, B.; McDowell, D.; and Muskins, P. (1990). Medical student attitudes toward AIDS, homosexual, and intravenous drug abusing patients: A re-evaluation in New York City. *Psychosomatics, 31*, 426–433.

Meisenhelder, J., and LaCharite, C. (1989). Fear of contagion: A stress response to Acquired Immuno Deficiency Syndrome. *Adv. Nursing Sci., 11*, 29–38.

Merrill, J.; Laux, L.; and Thornby, J. (1989). AIDS and student attitudes. *South. Med. J., 4*, 426–432.

Miller, J. (1976). *Toward a new psychology of women*. Boston: Beacon Press.

Miller, S. (1975). Introduction: The present cultural crisis and the need for a humanistic medicine. In S. Miller, et al., *Dimensions of humanistic medicine*. San Francisco: Institute for the Study of Humanistic Medicine.

Mizrahi, T. (1986). *Getting rid of patients: Contradictions in the socialization of physicians*. New Brunswick: Rutgers University Press.

Montgomery, C. (1991). Caring vs. curing. *Common Boundary, 9*, 37–40.

Moyers, B. (1993). *Healing and the mind*. New York: Doubleday.

Murphy, P. (1992). Empathy of intensive care nurses and critical care family needs. *Heart and Lung, 21*, 1.

Novak, D.; Volk, G.; Drossman, D.; and Lipkin, M. (1993). Medical interviewing and interpersonal skills teaching in U.S. medical schools. *JAMA, 269*, 2101–2105.

Olmstead, M. (1993). A doctor's story. *Mirabella*, Aug., p. 131.

Parke, R. (1969). Effectiveness of punishment as an interaction of intensity, timing, agent nurturance, and cognitive structuring. *Child Development, 40*, 211–235.

Phillips, E. (1988). *Patient compliance: New light on health delivery systems in medicine and psychotherapy*. Lewiston, N.Y.: Hans Huber.

Quill, T. (1983). Partnerships in patient care: A contractual approach. *Ann. Int. Med., 98*, 228–234.

————. (1989). Recognizing and adjusting to barriers in doctor–patient communication. *Ann. Int. Med., 111*, 51–57.

Remen, N. (1975). *The masculine principle, the feminine principle and humanistic medicine*. San Francisco: Institute for the Study of Humanistic Medicine.

Riffenburgh, R. (1974). Active Listening in the medical interview. *Post-grad. Med., 55*, 91–93.

Robinson, D. (1973). Ten noted doctors answer ten tough questions. *Parade*, July 15.

Rogers, C. (1951). *Client-centered therapy*. Boston: Houghton Mifflin.

Roter, D., and Hall, J. (1992). *Doctors talking with patients/Patients talking with doctors*. Westport, Conn.: Auburn House.

Roter, D.; Hall, J.; and Katz, N. (1988). Patient–physician communication: A descriptive summary of the literature. *Parent Ed. and counseling, 12*, 99–119.

Rowland-Morin, P., and Carroll, J. G. (1990). Verbal communication skills and patient satisfaction. *Evaluation and the Health Professions, 13*, 2.

Ruderman, W.; Weinblatt, E.; Goldberg, J.; and Chauhary, B. D. (1984). Psychosocial influences on mortality after myocardial infarction. *NEJM, 31*, 552–559.

Sackeim, H. (1993). Effects of stimulus intensity and electrode placement efficacy and cognitive effects of electroconvulsive therapy. *NEJM, 328*.

Shapiro, R.; Simpson, D.; and Lawrence, S. (1989). A survey of sued and nonsued physicians and suing patients. *Arch. Int. Med. 149*, 2190–2196.

Siegel, B. (1986). *Love, medicine, and miracles*. New York: Harper & Row.

Simmons, J., and Mares, W. (1983). *Working together*. New York: Alfred A. Knopf.

Solomon, G.; Tomoshok, L.; O'Leary, A.; and Zich, J. (1987). An intensive psychoimmunologic study of long-surviving persons with AIDS. *Ann. N.Y. Acad. Sci., 496*, 647–655.

Solomon, J. (1990). AIDS and caregivers. In R. Kus, ed., *Keys to caring: Assisting your gay and lesbian clients*. Boston: Alyson.

Spencer, F. (1990). The vital role in medicine of commitment to the patient. *Am. Coll. Surg. Bull.*, *75*, 6–19.

Svarstad, B. (1974). The doctor–patient encounter: An observational study of communication and outcome. Ph.D. diss., University of Wisconsin, Madison.

————. (1976). Physician–patient communication and patient conformity with medical advice. In D. Mechanic, ed., *The growth of bureaucratic medicine*. New York: Wiley.

Szasz, T., and Hollander, M. (1956). A contribution to the philosophy of medicine: The basic models of the doctor–patient relationship. *Arch. Int. Med.*, *97*. 585–592.

Treadway, J. (1983). Patient satisfaction and the content of general practice consultations. *J. Royal Coll. Gen. Pract.*, *33*, 769–771.

Waitzkin, H. (1984). doctor–patient communication: Clinical implications of social scientific research. *JAMA*, *252*, 2441–2446.

Zaiss, C., and Gordon, T. (1993). *Sales effectiveness training*. New York: Dutton.

Index

About the Authors

THOMAS GORDON, Ph.D., is President of Effectiveness Training International, Solana Beach, California. He is the creator of the pioneering program, Parent Effectiveness Training (P.E.T.), now taught in 37 countries. His training program for managers is used by the most successful companies in the United States.

W. STERLING EDWARDS, M.D., is Professor and Chairman Emeritus of the Department of Surgery at the University of New Mexico School of Medicine. He is the author of numerous books and publications in the medical field.